Medicine & Compassion

Publisher's Acknowledgment

THE PUBLISHER GRATEFULLY ACKNOWLEDGES the kind help of the Hershey Family Foundation in sponsoring the publication of this book

MEDICINE & COMPASSION

A Tibetan Lama's Guidance for Caregivers

Chokyi Nyima Rinpoche
with David R. Shlim, M.D.

Translated by Erik Pema Kunsang

Foreword by Harvey Fineberg and Donald Fineberg

Wisdom Publications • Boston

Wisdom Publications, Inc.
199 Elm Street
Somerville MA 02144 USA
www.wisdompubs.org

Library of Congress Cataloging-in-Publication Data
Nyima, Chokyi, 1951-
    Medicine & compassion : a Tibetan Lama's guidance for caregivers /
    Chokyi Nyima Rinpoche ; with David R. Shlim ; translated by Erik
    Pema Kunsang. foreword by Harvey Fineberg and Donald Fineberg.

    p. cm.
    ISBN 0-86171-478-4 (hardcover : alk. paper)
    1. Medicine—Religious aspects—Buddhism. 2. Compassion—
Religious aspects—Buddhism. 3. Buddhism—China—Tibet—Doctrines.
I. Shlim, David R. II. Title. III. Title: Medicine and compassion.
  BQ4570.M4N95 2004
  294.3'3661—dc22

        2004012882

First Edition
09 08 07 06 05 04
6   5   4   3   2   1

Wisdom Publications' books are printed on acid-free paper and meet the
guidelines for the permanence and durability set by the Council of Library
Resources.

Cover design by Rick Snizik
Interior design by Gopa & Ted2, Inc. Set in Fairfield LH Light 10.5/16.

Printed in the United States of America.

The bottom line is that being a kind, aware, and relaxed person doesn't require the belief in past and future lives, or the law of karma. It has to do with how we conduct ourselves, how we train our own minds. When we do it in the right way, all good qualities start to manifest from our mind, and all negative traits begin to grow less and less. The whole spiritual path is contained within just that.

—Chokyi Nyima Rinpoche

In an absolute sense, compassion is the awakened nature of the mind.

—Dilgo Khyentse Rinpoche

This book is dedicated to the memory of Tulku Urgyen Rinpoche, Chokyi Nyima Rinpoche's compassionate and accomplished father, who embodied every quality described in this book. He remains an inspiration.

The leaf on the cover is from the Bodhi tree, a large shade tree commonly found in Nepal and India. It was a Bodhi tree that sheltered the Buddha as he meditated and attained enlightenment. In Buddhist philosophy the leaf symbolizes loving-kindness.

Table of Contents

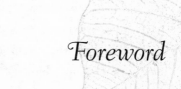

Foreword

"A physician shall be dedicated to providing competent medical care, with compassion and respect for human dignity and rights."—The first principle of the Code of Medical Ethics of the American Medical Association

Every doctor knows what it takes to become technically *competent*: learn more about scientific advances and the latest, successful drugs and procedures. How many physicians, however, have any sense of how to become more *compassionate*? Are some simply more inclined than others to be compassionate? Is it how they are born? Can you develop compassion in the same sense that you acquire other knowledge and skills that make up the craft of medicine?

The thesis of this exceptional book answers clearly: the conscientious physician *can* learn compassion. It can be done. A remarkable American physician, David Shlim, has done it. More importantly, he and his coauthor, the Tibetan lama Chokyi Nyima Rinpoche, describe how you can as well. Their approach to compassion in medicine emerged from their twenty-year relationship and derives from the philosophy of Tibetan Buddhism. It would be a mistake, however, to think that only an adherent of Buddhism could gain from reading, reflecting, and acting on this book's ideas. Beyond a statement of philosophy, this work provides practical guidance to anyone who seeks to become more compassionate.

Michelangelo was said to sculpt by liberating the figure within the marble. In similar fashion, Chokyi Nyima Rinpoche teaches here that compassion lies within each of us and emerges after removing the stumbling blocks of greed, anger, and ignorance. This requires effort and the mastery of technique, but compassion itself is not a technique. Compassion arises together with being a complete, understanding, and open person. In contemporary psychological terms, a focused intention to develop compassion takes advantage of the principles of cognitive consonance. Equipped with the knowledge of how to tap into your compassion, and acting on this understanding, you bring this feeling into your work and into your life. Your personal growth and professional depth go hand in hand.

The same qualities of mind that foster compassion—tolerating uncertainty, moment-to-moment awareness, openness to new information—can also engender better clinical decision-making. Compassion promotes competence. Compassionate physicians stay better focused on the true needs of their patients while taking full advantage of expert knowledge in treating them. In this way, compassion directly expresses "patient-centered" care, a key constituent of high-quality health care. Indeed, this concept was identified as a major dimension of quality in a 2001 report by the Institute of Medicine, *Crossing the Quality Chasm: A New Health System for the 21st Century.*

Medicine and Compassion reminds us that a compassionate physician copes better than one who is not. Compassion not only produces better care for the patient, it also strengthens the physician's ability to engage the difficult clinical situations of the terminally ill patient, the demanding patient, or the frustrated patient. Strengthening our compassion reminds us, too, of the motivation that led many to choose a career in medicine. In the face of multiple demands on doctors today, such reminders are more welcome than ever.

HARVEY V. FINEBERG, M.D., PH.D.
President, Institute of Medicine of the National Academies
Washington D.C.

DONALD E. FINEBERG, M.D.
Psychiatrist
Santa Fe, New Mexico

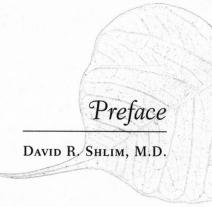

Preface

DAVID R. SHLIM, M.D.

M EDICINE AND COMPASSION—I don't think I ever heard those words spoken together in medical school." This comment from a friend, as I began to put this book together, alerted me to just how foreign a concept training in compassion might be. I had been living in Nepal for the past fifteen years running the world's busiest destination travel clinic. I had also been studying Tibetan Buddhism, and I had discovered that there is a body of knowledge on cultivating compassion that could greatly benefit a motivated caregiver.

In this book, Chokyi Nyima Rinpoche, a Tibetan lama who is the head of a large monastery in Nepal, presents a vision of kind, compassionate, and wise caregivers, and how we could train to be more like that. The book is timely, as it presents an antidote to the current climate in medicine that is dominated by high technology and an increased intrusion in medical care by financial considerations. Compassion for the patient, when considered at all, is assumed to already be present within the medical encounter simply because the purpose of the encounter is to try to make someone feel better or live longer. Even were a physician inspired to be more overtly compassionate, or able to handle difficult patients and situations with more grace, there is nowhere to go to develop that capacity.

A young physician just out of training once met Chokyi Nyima Rinpoche in Nepal. She asked him, "When I start out each day, I really want to help people, but by the end of the day I don't want to take care of anyone else. I've had it. Why is that?"

Chokyi Nyima Rinpoche replied, "Because you have not yet reached complete enlightenment. But it's very good that you start out each day wanting to help people."

This book is a guide for those who would start out each day wanting to help others, providing methods to both increase the desire and capacity to help while at the same time decreasing the effort required. The book describes what Buddhists call enlightenment, and demonstrates how such a state allows one to offer greater compassion with fewer limitations.

The philosophy of Tibetan Buddhism is based on the cultivation of compassion. Within Buddhism compassion is defined as the heartfelt desire to relieve the suffering of others. The method for training in compassion is based on recognizing that all beings have the capacity for compassion, and this capacity can be expanded and stabilized through training, resulting in more compassion with less effort. In other words, compassion is our natural state, so training in compassion is simply allowing our natural compassion to grow forth.

There is no question that the training works. The Dalai Lama is just one of hundreds of living examples within the Tibetan tradition who embody profound compassion and inspire it in others. Thousands of Tibetans over the past thousand years have taken these teachings to heart and achieved unshakable compassion and wisdom. Although these methods are just now being introduced to a wider Western audience, they have a long and proven history. This is not New Age stuff.

Caregivers typically approach the goal of being more compassionate toward patients by developing techniques—for better interviews, for increased empathy, or for more appropriate responses in difficult situations. However, many caregivers find that increased compassionate involvement exacts a burdensome emotional toll—the closer they get to a patient, the harder it becomes to cope with the patient's suffering. Ultimately, even the most compassionate caregivers may reach a point where they can no longer care as deeply or find meaning in their work. Thus, it is especially fortuitous that the Tibetan Buddhist method allows compassion to increase while simultaneously becoming more effortless. True compassion feels good for both the giver and the receiver. Rather than increasing stress, it relieves stress.

Training in compassion, however, does require some effort. Most people agree that doctors are more skillful at treating people after twenty years of practice than they are when they first start out. Like the study of medicine itself, the cultivation of compassion can become a lifelong pursuit, with continued improvement throughout. Readers of this book should approach training in compassion the way they might approach learning to play the piano. You can't hope to go to a weekend seminar in piano playing and come away a concert pianist. Just like expertise at the piano, increased compassion is a result of consistent daily practice, not a sudden burst of inspiration.

The teachings within this book represent the first time that a Tibetan lama has specifically tailored Tibetan Buddhist philosophy to the needs of Western doctors, nurses, and other caregivers. The teachings are presented in simpler language than is usual, but the range of philosophy that is covered encompasses the full scope of Tibetan Buddhism. You could study Tibetan Buddhism for the rest of your life, and still find that what you are learning has been already outlined in this book.

The book is divided into three sections. The first section gives an overview of human nature, compassion, and the problems that caregivers face in maintaining compassion. The second section provides instruction in how to specifically train in techniques that increase one's capacity for compassion—allowing compassion to be both more vast and more effortless. The third section addresses specific types of difficult patients and situations and gives practical advice on how to deal with irritable and angry patients, dying patients, and the parents of dying children.

For those who come to recognize their value, these teachings are said to be like pure gold. Gold, however, doesn't exist in its pure form in the ground. It has to be dug up, separated, and melted to achieve the form that we appreciate. Similarly, the teachings need to be studied, reflected upon, and then applied in one's daily life in order to be of practical value.

Everything we accomplish in this life begins with the first impulse to achieve something new. Simply feeling the desire to be more compassionate is the first, powerful step toward achieving this goal. Starting each day with the desire to help others, we may eventually be able to finish the day with the same wish. This book is dedicated to those who would discover their own pure-gold compassionate nature and use it for the benefit of all beings.

Acknowledgments

I would like to thank Chokyi Nyima Rinpoche for his unfailing support of this project. The gratitude that I have for him can hardly be overstated. He has patiently shared his insights into consciousness and compassion with me over a period of twenty years. In response to my request that he teach a course for medical professionals, he didn't hesitate despite an already extraordinarily busy schedule. His rationale for making time to teach doctors and nurses is that he felt that he could teach a relatively small number of people who in turn might be inspired to help relieve the suffering of thousands of people.

I would also like to pay special tribute to Erik Hein Schmidt, who translates under the Tibetan name Erik Pema Kunsang. The most skillful and beautiful teachings in the Tibetan language would be absolutely without value to English-speaking people without the help of skilled translators. Erik is among the best in the world, and through him the insights of Tibetan Buddhism are spreading to new audiences.

My thanks to Wisdom Publications for seeing the importance of this book in bringing Tibetan Buddhist philosophy into the practical realm of helping caregivers be more compassionate.

I'd like to thank my wife, Jane, and my children, Matthew and Anna Tara, for continuing to believe in the value of this project, despite taking five years to come to fruition in this book.

There are also the many great Tibetan masters who, through the circumstances of becoming physically ill, required the care of a Western doctor. I was privileged to treat these lamas, and to receive instruction on Buddhist philosophy and meditation in return. Although there are too many to list, I would like to especially thank Chogye Trichen Rinpoche, Dilgo Khyentse Rinpoche, Chokling Rinpoche, and Tsoknyi Rinpoche.

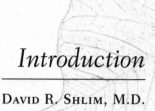

Introduction

David R. Shlim, M.D.

Halfway through my first year of residency I found myself wishing that a patient would die so that I could go back to sleep. The medical training I was undergoing often required that I stay awake for thirty-six hours at a time. On this particular night I had been up working until 4:00 A.M., my twenty-second hour on duty. I had just fallen asleep in the windowless on-call room when the phone jarred me awake and I was summoned to the emergency room to admit a new patient, my seventh of the night. I had come to understand why hospital slang for a patient to be admitted was a "hit." I staggered toward the emergency room like a boxer in the late rounds of a losing bout. I suddenly had the thought that if the patient died before I got there, I could go back to sleep, rather than spend the next two to three hours talking to, examining, and writing notes on the new patient. It was a happy thought at the time.

The patient in question, a woman in her fifties, did not die. She had stiff bleached hair and puffy cheeks streaked with mascara-stained tears. She wept through a litany of pains, none of which were due to any physical illness. If someone had walked in on us during those predawn hours, it would have been difficult to discern who was more unhappy—the patient or the doctor-in-training, who was unsuccessfully trying to be compassionate.

I had been highly motivated by compassion as a child, always trying to help others who were hurt or wild animals that needed care. My father was a doctor and a good example of a compassionate physician. But compassion had been slowly leeched from my system during my years of medical training, replaced by the persistent thought: *it's either them or me.* The patients, whose suffering was supposed to be my main concern, had become instead the source of *my* suffering—by preventing my sleep, by having emotional needs I couldn't meet, and by failing to get better while I was taking care of them. "Patients can always hurt you more," is one of the main rules in *The House of God,* an insightful novel about a doctor's first year of training at a major medical center.

I hadn't forgotten about compassion, but it now seemed like a luxury that I couldn't afford. Fatigue ruled my waking moments. "For many residents," wrote a doctor who studied resident training, "fatigue cultivates anger, resentment, and bitterness, rather than kindness, compassion, or empathy." An overwhelming amount of medical training is crammed into a few years. The constant pressure to perform under adverse circumstances helps create mentally tough doctors who can function through crisis and exhaustion. I began to wonder, however, when and how compassion for patients is encouraged in a doctor's career. If medical training itself was undermining whatever compassion I had brought to the study of medicine, when was I going to become the kind, compassionate, and wise physician I hoped to be?

If compassion is indeed valued in medicine, it's not clear when it is emphasized in medical training. Applicants to medical school are selected mainly on the basis of academic achievement rather than a proven desire to help others. Once enrolled in medical school, students are overwhelmed by the need to learn the basic science that underpins medical care, and later by the pressures of actual patient care and the fear of making a mistake. If they spend more time comforting each patient, they are often accused by their supervising resident of not being efficient. Once residency training starts, efficiency is the most highly valued skill. Demonstrating that you can manage the workload is far more important than showing that you can be compassionate.

After years of training in this setting, doctors tend to remain focused on the mechanics of medical care—diagnosis and treatment—and rarely spend much time imagining what it feels like to be a patient under their own care. Only after their training is completed do doctors finally have the opportunity to discern their own values in relation to compassion—giving what they can while at the same time protecting themselves from becoming overwhelmed by emotionally difficult situations.

It's ironic that this lack of overt compassion in medicine comes at a time when medicine can do more for a patient than at any time in history. Major advances of the past fifty years include antibiotics, anti-inflammatories, sophisticated non-invasive diagnostic capabilities, minimally invasive surgical techniques, immunization against a wide variety of diseases, kidney dialysis, open-heart surgery, and organ transplantation. Despite these remarkable achievements, few people seem as happy as they should be with the way medicine is practiced. Surveys show that doctors are less satisfied with their careers than ever before. Patients often complain about their medical care, and the people who manage healthcare systems throw up their hands at making medicine affordable or universally available. A piece of the puzzle is missing, and that missing piece may be compassion.

The lack of an overt sense of compassion in medicine may actually be due to, rather than in spite of, recent technical advances. By utilizing the potent arsenal at their fingertips, doctors often help patients feel and get better. Doctors take for granted that by alleviating their patients' symptoms they are expressing compassion, and are confused when patients don't appear to be as appreciative as they should be.

Compassion is assumed to be present in the medical encounter—what we could call "de facto compassion." Patients look for reassurance and kindness from their physicians, but what they receive often feels impersonal. The doctor projects an attitude that can be expressed as: "Of course I care for you—I'm caring for you aren't I?"

Some of the difficulty in defining compassionate care stems from a lack of comfort with the word compassion itself. The word compassion is not in medical dictionaries. In a standard dictionary, compassion is primarily defined as "to suffer with." Taking this definition literally and simply sharing the suffering of patients would not seem to help either patients or physicians. The definition of the word compassion also connotes sympathy, which medical professionals avoid because it appears condescending toward patients. Therefore, the word compassion rarely appears in the medical literature. Words currently in vogue include "humanism" and "caring."

Doctors fear that if they open themselves up to the emotions of their patients, they will be overwhelmed. They feel that they need to distance themselves from the pain, loneliness, and fear that many patients are suffering. If they identify too closely with their patients, they run the risk of emotional exhaustion. Emotional exhaustion can interfere with their ability to make clear decisions, so they try to maintain an objective distance, a distance that the patient interprets as not caring enough. In this way, doctors have built an emotional Catch-22 into the practice of medicine: the only way they feel they can care more for patients is by not caring too much.

The need to increase the connection between doctors and patients has not gone unnoticed by medical schools. Medical school administrators have designed courses to help young doctors better handle difficult clinical situations. Most of these courses are aimed at first- and second-year students who haven't yet had much patient contact and thus have little real responsibility. The courses focus on developing empathy—an understanding of how the patient is feeling. The courses also teach techniques that can be employed to help deal with angry, depressed, or grieving patients.

Some medical students may be inspired to apply these principles to their patients once they reach the wards. However, the environment of constant pressure to get the work done soon eclipses their impulses toward compassion. This compassion-stifling milieu has been dubbed "the hidden curriculum," because it conveys the unspoken message— to just get on with it—that students actually receive during their medical training.

Students who allow themselves to care more deeply about their patients in this unsupportive atmosphere eventually find that they need to erect an emotional barrier to protect themselves. With no coaching or mentoring on how to train in compassion and cope with the suffering of patients, they find that they are emotionally unequipped to handle the sheer volume of suffering they encounter. When the student confesses to having reached this point, their teachers and colleagues then confirm to them that this is why they themselves keep an emotional distance from patients—they can indeed "always hurt you more." What's missing is a way to help doctors offer greater compassion with less effort, to confront emotional trauma without having a negative impact on their own mental health.

We are at our most compassionate when we are most relaxed. When the focus is off our own emotions, anger, or irritability, we are naturally more open to the concerns of others. However, caring more deeply while at the same time feeling more relaxed is not natural to most of us. To achieve this desirable goal, some training is necessary. The idea that we can increase our capacity for compassion through training is not yet an accepted concept in medical education—nor in any Western educational setting. The main goal of this book is to demonstrate that there is a highly successful 2500-year-old tradition of training in compassion that can be applied to the Western medical setting.

We tend to think that you either have compassion or you don't. We aren't certain about where compassion comes from, so we use it sparingly, reserving it for select situations. We feel that compassion is like a battery—once it's turned on it will be steadily drained until it eventually has to be recharged. We even speak of holidays as a way to "recharge our batteries." But like a rechargeable battery, the ability to achieve a full charge diminishes with time. Eventually, the lack of ability to continue caring for others and find meaning in one's work may end the health professional's career, a phenomenon called burnout.

I was approaching burnout when I decided to move to Kathmandu in 1983. I had worked in family practice for eighteen months in a small logging town in northern California, but I didn't fit into the small-town life there. For the next four years I worked as an emergency room physician in Portland, Oregon, my hometown. Emergency medicine appealed to me because of the clear demarcation between work and time off, which allowed me to take rock climbing trips for weeks at a time. The adrenaline-charged moments of tension and teamwork while caring for critically ill patients in the emergency room generated some of the same feelings I had while I was climbing. However, the twelve-hour night shifts eventually led to a feeling of persistent jet lag on my days off. Moreover, the nighttime emergency room was at the center of a continuing battle with the unsolved social problems of our society. The automatic doors were designed to slide open for the beaten, homeless, mentally ill, violent—or all of the above. Although I cared about these people, I couldn't solve their underlying problems in the setting of the emergency room. It was a Band-Aid approach to an overwhelming social neglect. After six years, I was still waiting for the practice of medicine to feel gratifying.

During these six years I traveled to Nepal three times, working in a small rescue post near the base of Mt. Everest for three months at a time, taking care of mountain climbers, trekkers, and local people. I met the people who had written the books that had inspired me to seek adventure in the Himalayas—Sir Edmund Hillary, Reinhold Messner, Galen Rowell. I faced major medical problems alone in a stone hut at 14,000 feet in a remote Himalayan valley. For the first time I felt a direct connection between the effort I made on behalf of patients and how much I felt appreciated.

During my third stay in the mountains, I finally faced up to the fact that I was disenchanted with emergency medicine back home. I didn't know what to do next—I couldn't volunteer to stay year-round in a summer yak-herding village (even the Sherpas didn't live there year-round), and I didn't want to return to the emergency room. It was at that point that I heard about the CIWEC Clinic in Kathmandu—a Western-run clinic that had been established in 1982 to care for foreigners in Nepal (CIWEC stands for Canadian International Water and Energy Consultants—the aid group that put up the funds to start the clinic initially). My stint in the mountains finished as winter approached. I walked three days to the airstrip at Lukla and flew to Kathmandu. I met the medical director of the CIWEC Clinic, was offered a job, and started work in August 1983. I planned to work there for one or two years, but I ended up staying for fifteen.

The CIWEC Clinic was the world's first destination travel clinic—the first clinic to concentrate the care of foreigners in a developing country into a single institution. It is still the world's busiest. Travelers who appeared at the clinic door were often desperately ill and incredibly relieved to find Western faces and a high standard of medical care.

In my second year in Nepal I started volunteering to see monks at a Tibetan monastery, holding sick call on Saturdays. The head of the monastery was Chokyi Nyima Rinpoche. He was born in 1950, the same year the Chinese started invading eastern Tibet. He was recognized at eighteen months of age as the reincarnation of the head of a monastery northeast of Lhasa. As Chinese influence and atrocities spread westward toward Lhasa, intolerance of the monastic community reached murderous levels. Tibetans started to emigrate out of Tibet into Nepal and India, and Chokyi Nyima Rinpoche's family left Tibet in 1958. The following year, a mass emigration of hundreds of thousands of Tibetans took place just after the Dalai Lama had to flee to avoid capture by the Chinese in Lhasa.

Chokyi Nyima Rinpoche (*Rinpoche* is an honorific title meaning "precious") received monastic training at Rumtek Monastery in Sikkim, India, under the direct supervision of the head of his lineage, the sixteenth Karmapa.* Chokyi Nyima Rinpoche trained at Rumtek for eleven years. After spending his final year as the Karmapa's personal attendant, he was instructed by his teacher to build a monastery in the Kathmandu Valley and make himself available to the growing numbers of Westerners who were becoming interested in Tibetan Buddhism.

Chokyi Nyima Rinpoche was in his early thirties, a year younger than myself, when I first met him in Nepal in 1984. He lived on the top floor of his monastery, a massive white structure overlooking the Boudhanath Stupa, one of the most important Buddhist pilgrimage sites in the world. The monastery housed about eighty monks at the time (now over 250). His private bedroom opened into a large greeting area. Each Saturday when I went out to hold my clinic for the monks, I'd climb four flights of stairs to see him. We'd sit on handcarved wooden couches at one end of his greeting room and have tea,

---

* There are four main lineages in Tibetan Buddhism. His Holiness the Dalai Lama is associated primarily with the Geluk lineage. The Karmapa is the head of the main branch of the Kagyu lineage. The other two lineages are Nyingma and Sakya.

chatting about current events. He often invited me back to have lunch with him after I saw the monks.

In Chokyi Nyima Rinpoche I encountered a maturity, wisdom, and compassion that I had never observed before. Although we were the same age, I began to see him as a father figure, someone who was always ready and able to give caring and useful advice. His advice was based on Buddhist philosophy, and I started to see how the Buddhist viewpoint could help me function more easily in difficult and painful situations. Learning about Tibetan Buddhism directly from someone who had mastered the tradition both philosophically and experientially made it seem remarkably scientific and clear.

The many Tibetan lamas I met in Nepal embodied a rich and courageous form of compassion. They were able to offer kindness and wisdom to everyone. They faced challenging situations with equanimity. Even when their own lives were threatened by terminal illness, their calm acceptance, and their compassion toward others, never wavered. They remained kind, calm, and completely unafraid even at the end of life.

I was once asked to see a Tibetan lama in the end stages of liver cancer who was staying in a house about a twenty minutes' drive from my clinic. It was the end of the day, when the normally congested streets congeal even more into a barely flowing river of people, animals, smoke-belching trucks, cars, and motorcycles. I was greeted at the door by anxious monks who ushered me into the lama's bedroom. His eyes were a deep yellow color with jaundice, and he had a hugely distended abdomen that bulged upward toward his lungs, making breathing difficult. He thanked me for coming and told me that it must have been difficult to drive through the traffic at that time of day. Although he was in severe pain and could barely breathe, he was genuinely concerned that I had had to face some traffic to come see him. He died the next morning.

In addition to taking care of members of the monastic community, I began to see newly arrived Tibetan refugees, mainly young people who had trekked over the Himalayan range through 20,000-foot passes to escape the hardship of Chinese rule in Tibet. If they were unlucky enough to get caught in a storm, they didn't have the luxury of retreat, because they would be arrested and often tortured if caught trying to return from their escape attempt. One consequence of pushing on for several days with poor clothing through terrible storms was severe frostbite. As I cared for them—many required amputation of fingers and toes and one to two months to recover—I listened to heartbreaking stories of imprisonment and torture at the hands of the Chinese authorities in Tibet. No matter how horrible the story, almost every one of the refugees talked about it with calm detachment and little apparent bitterness.

One story that still haunts me was told by a young man in his twenties who was imprisoned for putting up posters against Chinese rule in Tibet. Every night in the deep cold of winter he would be stripped naked and taken to the roof of the prison. He was then drenched in freezing water and left tied to a post outside through the long bitter night at over 12,000 feet in altitude. He would very nearly freeze to death each night, but in the morning he would be taken back to his cell and allowed to warm up. He would then face the same treatment again the next night.

I also met an older Tibetan doctor who had undergone severe hardship and starvation in a Chinese prison for almost twenty years. I asked him if he had any bitterness toward the Chinese. He told me, "The suffering that I went through in prison was due to my own karma, and now it is finished. If I killed a Chinese soldier, it would not undo the suffering that I have already gone through and would only create the cause for me to undergo more suffering in the future. So what would be the point?"

All of this contact with Tibetans made me yearn to visit Tibet and see for myself the country that nurtured people with such remarkable strength and spirituality. In 1987 I finally crossed the Himalayas by road onto the high Tibetan plateau.

The ruins of thousands of monasteries were like poorly healed scars on this otherwise barely touched landscape. The Chinese had tried to purge Tibet of its Buddhist foundation, and—at least in regard to build-ings—had been over 90 percent successful. In addition, virtually all of the great Buddhist masters of Tibet had fled, been imprisoned, or killed.

The trip to Tibet made me even more appreciative of the contact I had with the lamas who lived in Nepal. The kindness and generosity that I felt from my closest teachers engendered a growing gratitude and appreciation for what they had to teach. Striving to emulate these extraordinary examples of wisdom and compassion made me more committed to my meditation practice. Over time, I became aware that my encounters with patients were changing in positive ways. I was able to create an environment that allowed patients to more easily say what they needed to say. Encouraging and appropriate words arose more effortlessly. I found I had more patience for irritable and angry people. I could help comfort severely ill or dying patients more easily. In other words, I had found a way to train in being the kind of doctor I had always wanted to be.

I experienced this not as an overnight revelation but as a gradual change. It confirmed for me that it was possible to train in being a kinder and more compassionate physician. This realization led to a desire to try to organize a conference on medicine and compassion for a Western audience. I mentioned the idea to Chokyi Nyima Rin-poche, who agreed that he would teach such a course to doctors and nurses if I could arrange it someday. I nurtured the idea for many years, until I finally moved back to the United States, to Jackson Hole, Wyoming, in 1998.

I decided that the medicine and compassion course would be struc-
tured like a traditional medical conference. Attendees would receive
continuing medical education credit, a syllabus, and would sit at tables
and chairs—classroom style—rather than on cushions on the floor as
is traditional at many Buddhist teachings. I created brochures and
mailed 50,000 randomly to doctors and nurses. I avoided promoting
the conference to doctors and nurses who were already deeply
involved in Buddhism; to see whether Tibetan Buddhism had something to offer everyday working doctors and nurses, I needed to test
the concept on a naïve audience.

The first course, "Medicine and Compassion," was held in September 2000 and drew sixty-five doctors and nurses. The second
course, "Medicine and Wisdom," drew ninety people in June 2002.
The teachings presented in this book are edited from the transcripts
of both conferences. Chokyi Nyima Rinpoche's teachings distill the
wisdom of Tibetan Buddhism into simple language tailored to the
needs of the caring professions. However, the relevance of the book
is not limited to the practice of medicine. The teachings here can also
be read as a remarkably accessible introduction to the most profound
Tibetan Buddhist concepts.

Those who practice medicine often feel that the main obstacle to
bringing more compassion to their work is that they don't have enough
time. Chokyi Nyima Rinpoche makes it clear that one can cultivate a
compassionate attitude—a genuine motivation to ease suffering—that
will be evident in one's demeanor regardless of the time constraints.
By training in compassion, one naturally becomes more relaxed, which
leads to clearer thinking and more energy to expend on solving a
patient's problems.

If one is able to bring a compassionate attitude into the exam room,
the patient can feel it and will be better able to communicate what
they are really worried about. When the patient can truly open up,

the doctor can do a better job of meeting the patient's needs. This leads to a greater sense of gratification on the part of the doctor at the end of the day. By focusing on compassion, people who design health-care systems may begin to help provide what patients actually require to ease suffering, rather than getting caught up in plans to decrease costs and ration care. Focusing on compassion may even be one approach to the struggle that we here in America face to provide universally available and satisfying medical care.

The weeks leading up to the first course in September of 2000 were marked by a terrible drought in the American West. Fires were burning out of control in many states, and flames were visible in all directions from Jackson Hole, including a forest fire within Grand Teton National Park. Firefighters were overstretched and exhausted; experts said that the fires would only be brought under control by the onset of winter snows.

The day Chokyi Nyima Rinpoche flew into Jackson Hole for the medicine and compassion course it rained the entire day—the first rainfall in almost two months. It continued to rain another two days throughout the West, extinguishing fires and easing the burden on firefighters. Chokyi Nyima Rinpoche commented on the rains during the course: "These days, a lot of forest has been on fire in the United States, and now the rain of compassion is falling, which is quite wonderful. Now it is not just talk, but in actuality, the forests burning from the fire of anger are being subdued by the rain of compassion. The gentle rain of compassion is putting out the fires of anger."

Were everyone to cultivate the gentle rain of compassion, the fires of anger throughout the world might be subdued. Not just in talk, but in actuality. What better place to start than with the healing arts—the practice of medicine.

Prologue

CHOKYI NYIMA RINPOCHE

T HE PURPOSE OF THIS BOOK is to investigate how to combine compassion with the art of healing. How can we best combine these
two factors, and what would be the value of doing so? Compassion is
an attitude, a way of approaching the needs of others. People develop
many different attitudes in their lives, but the attitude that we call
compassion is the most noble and the most helpful for others. The fact
that compassion is important is commonly accepted. Affirming the
value of compassion has little to do with whether you consider yourself spiritual, or whether you choose to follow—or not—any particular religion.

In Buddhist philosophy, the cultivation of compassion receives special attention. Buddhist teachings refer to "the precious enlightened
attitude of benevolence." This precious enlightened attitude expresses
itself as a loving, considerate, and compassionate will to help others.
Does it make practical sense to try to cultivate kindness and compassion when the world appears to be so competitive? It might seem like
the prudent thing to do is to simply look out for your own interests or
the interests of those closest to you. If you think about it, however, the
situation in the world today, with all of its conflicts, makes it even
more urgent to study and train in compassion. For the main factor
that promotes peace and well-being is compassion.

My student Dr. David Shlim has meditated and studied for many years. He began to think that it could be beneficial to share what he has learned. He thought, "I am a doctor, and many doctors have the same feelings that I do. We like to serve others, and we would like to develop loving-kindness. The teachings about loving-kindness and wisdom are very clear and perfect in Buddhist philosophy." So he thought like this for a long time. And he kept asking me, "I would like you to provide teachings specifically for medical professionals about medicine and compassion. Will you do this someday?"

I know this topic is very important for doctors, so I made time to do this. How much this will help you or not, I can't say. I'm very pleased that you made the effort to obtain this book. What drew you to read this book? You naturally feel kindness toward those in your care, and you want to develop that kindness in yourself and others. That's a very, very good reason for you to want to read a book about medicine and compassion.

I wish that you may be happy and healthy, and that your wisdom and loving-kindness may increase like the waxing moon. This is my wish and my prayer.

OVERVIEW

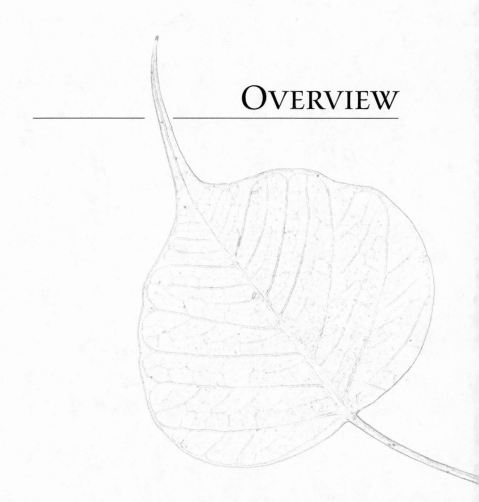

1

Human Nature

OVER THE LAST TWO HUNDRED YEARS, the world appears to have totally changed due to developments in science. It is now possible to travel great distances in a very short time. The practice of medicine has also benefited from scientific innovations. Surgery has improved dramatically, and diseases can now be cured that in the past were impossible to treat. If people from a couple of centuries ago suddenly arrived in our time, they would think that our modern inventions were a form of magic.

Although much of this development has been positive and helpful, some developments have been frightening and destructive. Massive genocides have occurred, and there is the constant threat of nuclear and bioterrorist attacks. Good and evil appear to flourish together. We need to investigate why.

The helpful, positive developments that we experience all derive from human intelligence. None of them just fall from the sky. The technological advances were not created by gods, nor were their destructive uses produced by the devil. Some people say that the gods create what is good, while all the harmful and abusive activity in the world is the work of the devil. In my view, it's not like that.

The helpful, positive developments in human civilization are a product of creative human intelligence. Likewise, destructive inventions also come from the human mind. If we examine any person's character closely, we can always find something kind and positive. If we look even more closely, we will discover that these compassionate qualities are intrinsic—they are inherently present in the mind of every person. In some people such feelings may be just a tiny seed, but they are still present.

At the same time, there is also an aggressive and potentially nasty side to most any human being. If we ask, "What is the nature of a given person?" the answer would be that each person is a mixture of positive and negative qualities. We sometimes experience spontaneous feelings of compassion toward others, while at other times we feel selfish and angry.

Any being capable of having experiences is called a *sentient being*. The fundamental quality of being able to experience is identical for each of us. To use an analogy, we could say that our basic nature is like water. Water has the inherent quality of being wet. Is it possible to find water that is not wet? Not a liquid? If you do find dry water, it is not called water any more. In addition, pure water appears sparklingly clear. However, we sometimes encounter water that is brown and muddy. When water is mixed with dirt it appears muddy, but pure water is still present. If we filter out the dirt, we will still have completely pure water. It's the same within ourselves. Our basic nature is very clear and clean, but it can appear to be muddy. Water is a convenient example, because we are all very familiar with the qualities of water.

We can combine the example with its meaning. Just like water has the quality of being an inherently clear liquid, our basic nature— called *mind* in Buddhist philosophy—has the property of being compassionate. While we may generally accept that this is true for any human being, we might not acknowledge that this is also true for every other sentient being. Yet even the most short-tempered, vicious animal that we can think of, such as a tiger or a leopard, always has someone that they care for, that they are happy to see again, that they love and protect. Perhaps you have seen movies of mother tigers and leopards tenderly caring for their babies, and teaching them how to care for themselves in the wild. If we look closely, we may find that all sentient beings are capable of compassion at some level.

The capacity for compassion is combined with the capacity for intelligence. These two aspects of our basic nature have incredible power and enormous potential. Human intelligence can lead to remarkably beneficial things. It can discover cures for disease, or vaccines that prevent infections in millions of people. Doctors now have the ability to reach inside the human body using scopes and imaging devices to cure problems without resorting to painful, invasive surgery.

There are other useful inventions as well, such as a machine that can carry four hundred people together through the air. At any one time, some passengers are eating, some are having conversations, some are asleep, and some are sitting on the toilet. Together they travel in one day from a place we call the East to a place we call the West. It's pretty incredible. What makes this possible? These inventions were not thought up by a computer. They weren't handed down from the sky by a god. Human intelligence—put to good use—is able to bring forth such beneficial inventions.

Human intelligence is the creator of these technological marvels. This fact is widely recognized, and has led to a lot of interest, and a lot of facilities where younger human beings can go to develop their intelligence. Western culture is oriented particularly around the kind of intelligence that can produce increasingly sophisticated material goods. But what about the other aspect of human minds—the capacity for being compassionate, and the qualities that go along with that? There appears to be less interest in these qualities, and fewer facilities set up to promote human compassion.

If we could have a better balance between the development of intelligence on one side and the development of a loving, compassionate frame of mind on the other, this world would be far more harmonious, far more at peace. I feel that it's critical at the present time to invest more effort into systematically developing love and compassion. Of course developing love and compassion is always important, but at present it is even more crucial. If we could advance the cultivation of love and compassion to the extent we have developed technological improvements, the entire world community would benefit immeasurably.

Buddhism defines compassion as the sincere wish to alleviate the suffering of another. This desire to alleviate another's pain includes not only their present experience of discomfort but also the cause of their suffering, the underlying reasons they are not well. This kind of genuine desire to make others feel better and not suffer is what compassion is all about.

Likewise, Buddhists define loving-kindness as the wish for another person both to be happy and to have the causes for happiness. It is the wish for another person's well-being. You not only want others to feel happier momentarily, you also want them to enjoy the causes for ongoing happiness.

Loving-kindness and compassion are feelings that are directed toward someone else. It feels natural to be loving and compassionate toward someone that we already know and like, such as our close friends, our children, or our parents. It is more difficult to feel love and compassion toward people we don't know, people that we have no prior relationship with. Even more difficult yet is to experience spontaneous love and compassion for people who harm us in some way, or for people who apparently dislike us or who criticize us.

You may have encountered someone in your life who has spoken badly of you in public, or who has tried to undermine you behind your back. This person may have been rude to you, or said cruel, hurtful words. It is incredibly difficult to feel compassion toward a person who treats you this way. According to the Buddha, we should aim at cultivating loving-kindness and compassion that knows no bounds, that is not limited to people we already know and like. However, we have already discovered that this type of boundless compassion does not come naturally. Unless we train ourselves, unless we put our heart into being that way, it will not develop. We need to train in developing our loving-kindness and compassion so that it eventually expresses itself without any prejudice or limitations.

This type of attitude may seem impossible to achieve, and it would be were it not for a key element in the Buddhist teachings that makes this goal possible. The Buddha taught that we should try to achieve a state of mind described as "emptiness suffused with compassion." *openness* Although "emptiness" is the most common translation, we can substitute the word "openness" for emptiness: the development of a feeling of openness that is suffused with compassion. For some people this may sound strange, while for others it may prove relatively easy to understand. This concept will be addressed in much greater detail later on, but for now simply recognize that we are not talking about a religious quality. Emptiness is something that is ultimately our basic nature.

For those who pursue training in compassion, intention and motivation are of central importance. The more pure, noble, and vast our intentions are, the better the outcome. When we initially express our intention to help others, we may not be able to visualize actually helping people on a vast scale. However, by simply aspiring to help others, no matter how many there are—countless others—sooner or later that wish can come true. By simply forming the wish or prayer, "May I help a huge number of others—not only people, but all beings," you will eventually succeed. Unfortunately, the same is true for evil desires. If you hold onto ill will for a long time, and continue to expand it into a huge aspiration, such as, "May I really harm others on a massive scale," then definitely at some point you will be able to do this.

A benevolent frame of mind can ease the suffering of other beings, and a malevolent frame of mind can cause immense suffering. Since you are reading this book, I assume you are interested in being able to relieve suffering. In order to be able to relieve suffering, and to avoid causing it, we need to investigate the causes of suffering in more detail.

2

The Causes of Suffering

CERTAIN TYPES OF SUFFERING are inevitable for us as human beings. It begins when we are born. Taking birth is not a simple thing for either the child or the mother. It can be incredibly painful and dangerous for both mother and child. If we survive birth and childhood, we grow up. Then there is a second problem—aging. The aging process can be unpleasant. We feel it gradually at first, as the body gets older and begins to lose some of its capacities and vitality. But when we get really old, it can be dreadful. At that point we are aware of all the activities we can no longer enjoy, and in addition we may suffer from constant discomfort or pain.

Then there is disease. A brief, mild illness we can stand. It's uncomfortable, but it's okay. However a severe illness is far more difficult to endure. Yet if it can be cured, it's not that bad. It's still better than a severe illness that is incurable. What if you become ill, and it never goes away? That can be unbearable. Which brings us to the fourth problem—having to die at some point. But death does not always come at the end of a protracted illness or at the end of a long life. Death can come without warning and at any point in our lives. The time of death is not fixed, but what is certain is that we must die some day. Exactly when and how we die is not certain. These four problems—birth, aging, sickness, and death—are shared by all human beings.

Human beings experience other types of suffering as well. Whether one is rich or poor, old or young, at least some sense of discomfort or dissatisfaction is always present. The discomfort stems from the feeling "I didn't get what I want." Each person has something he or she desires. It could be one main desire or many small desires. Desires often come one after another, like ripples on the water. The funny thing is that if you manage to achieve what you desire, another desire immediately pops into view. That's the problem. It's a big problem.

When you begin to desire something, by definition that means you haven't got it yet. While you are chasing that desire, there is a constant feeling of being unfulfilled. You are waiting and hoping for something that has yet to happen. And when you finally attain what you want, it is typically not as satisfying as you had hoped. Is it ever possible to say that we are permanently satisfied because we got what we wanted? That is the problem. This continuous cycle of desire and dissatisfaction makes people unhappy, and is itself a cause of suffering.

Suffering can result from a persistent feeling or worry that what we have is not good enough. We are unable to take joy in what we have, and instead remain focused on what we don't have. As long as we allow ourselves to be preoccupied in this way, we can never feel at ease. We are not able to say, "This is fine, I'm content."

If we don't train ourselves to relax a little bit, we'll never be happy. We'll never be at ease, even though outwardly it may appear that we have a happy life. We might look at someone living in luxurious surroundings eating exquisitely prepared food and assume they must be happy. But if we were to view these people from the inside, we might see that they are unable to genuinely appreciate life, that the comforts and pleasures cannot erase the underlying dissatisfaction. What does it help to be fabulously wealthy and own entire mountains if it doesn't really satisfy you? This feeling of being unfulfilled needs to be confronted; some education is necessary in order to be able to appreciate what you have. The goal is to be satisfied, to take delight in your life.

Everyone naturally strives to be healthy and happy. This in itself is not a problem. The problem is that we often look in the wrong place to satisfy this goal. As I have pointed out, simply acquiring more and more things does not solve the problem. How is it then accomplished? We need to investigate.

To begin with, we might ask who is it that wants to feel joy, to feel contentment? What actually experiences the joy or happiness that we are trying to get? It's our mind. Whenever our mind is at ease and feeling appreciative, then whatever we see, hear, smell, or touch is okay. It feels perfect.

The opposite is when our mind is disturbed—angry, afraid, proud, or jealous. When our emotions are in turmoil, that in itself is what we call suffering. When we are experiencing strong emotions, we don't perceive anything as okay, no matter how nice it may actually be. The objects around us are no longer pleasant, sounds are irritating, even the most expensive perfume is completely unenchanting. The finest Italian, French, or Chinese cuisine appears unappetizing. Even if you eat, the food tastes bland and uninteresting. The bottom line is that everything is changed when we have a negative frame of mind.

Why is that? Did the external objects change—what we see, hear, smell, and taste, and so forth? Normally it seems like that. If they had actually changed, then we wouldn't blame our emotional state, we'd blame the objects themselves. We'd say that it's not our fault that we feel awful. However, the objects themselves have not changed. When this mind becomes too emotionally disturbed, we experience everything as unpleasant. Our state of mind makes the difference. The opposite situation can also occur, wherein you experience your surroundings as pleasant and joyful, because your mind is relaxed and able to appreciate everything. If you don't cultivate the ability to appreciate, it makes no difference how exquisite your surroundings are.

Once we recognize suffering as something that stems from our mental state, we can begin to understand that there are many types of suffering on many levels. With diseases, some can be cured and some not. However, feeling emotionally ill at ease can always be cured if we know the right methods and apply them intelligently. From the Buddhist point of view, all types of mental pain, and ultimately physical suffering as well, can be traced back to a single cause, what is normally translated as *ignorance.* This may sound funny to you: ignorance is the root cause of physical disease and mental problems. Actually, it's a very profound statement.

Ignorance literally means "not knowing." What is it that is supposed to be known? We need to be able to recognize our basic nature—the original unconditioned state that lies at the very heart of every moment of consciousness. Whatever that nature is, it is not derived from religion or philosophy. It has to do simply with what is. Knowing the natural state is not a frame of mind. It's not a mode of perceiving. As a matter of fact, our basic nature is totally free of concepts. For without concepts, there is no platform—no basis—for emotional disturbance.

Let's say that we were able to experience and recognize our basic nature. We would still have a physical body made of bones, blood, flesh, and so forth. Having recognized and experienced our basic nature and become free of any conceptual attitudes, does that mean we wouldn't get sick any longer? No, it doesn't. The circumstances would still exist for our present physical body to become ill. But the emotional or psychological pain usually connected with becoming ill would have dissolved. The pain would not be as intense, and the suffering would not become overwhelming.

Another term that is used to describe awareness of the natural state is *natural mind*. When we are able to recognize natural mind, physical pain is not perceived in the same way. It still hurts, but it's not a big deal. There is no longer the huge burden of anxiety—we are simply concerned. Of course you feel and you notice, but it does not overwhelm you. It's not as intense as before. This is how it can be for someone who has grown used to recognizing their natural mind.

Let's examine the opposite situation. Imagine someone who cannot shed the thought, "I'm ill, it's horrible, I can't take it." They reproduce that thought over and over again, from moment to moment. They dwell on that thought so much that they truly believe, "I'm ill, it's horrible, I can't take it." Of course the person is physically ill, but the sense of helplessness and panic is a mental construct that is created on top of the illness.

That mental attitude is what makes the illness unbearable. Even when a person is not dealing with a physical illness, anxiety and fear can be magnified totally out of proportion. It can have very little to do with what is actually wrong in our lives, or what could actually happen. We worry so much that the fear itself becomes unbearable, even though the outcome we fear may never come to pass. If another worry comes along that is perceived as being more serious, the previous problem is forgotten. The new problem outweighs the first. Our attitude is what creates the sense of suffering. We could have an attitude that doesn't make a big deal out of our pain. An alternative attitude could be that we make it into a huge problem, even if it is actually quite minor. At that point, our problems become magnified so as to be almost unbearable. Everything has to do with attitude.

This is one place where the medical professional can really help. You can encourage the shift from a really negative attitude to a more positive, accepting attitude. You can encourage the patient, depending on the situation, "Have heart. We'll do what we can. You'll be okay. We can deal with this. Don't make yourself depressed, we're doing something about it." For if the patient gives up psychologically, treatment becomes much more difficult. Even with the right medicine and a very skilled doctor, treatment will not be very effective for someone who feels that all is hopeless. Psychologically giving up has a power that can affect the body. It's important for the patient to have hope, to think, "I want to get better quickly. I definitely want to live. I want to fight this disease. I want to be cured." This kind of strong motivation has a lot of power. It will affect the body. If the person has mental strength, it makes the body stronger and can make the medicine work better.

The point in this book is not merely to stress the importance of compassion. I think you sense this already or else you wouldn't be reading what I have to say. What we need to find out is how to actually *be* more compassionate. We know that compassion is important, but how do we actually make it more readily available? The first step is to really learn about suffering, to educate oneself about how illness feels. Human beings do suffer. It is not a painless process to live and grow old and die. There are many kinds of suffering, both physical and mental. Just applying medical knowledge cannot fully relieve the sense of suffering experienced by many patients.

If we happen to know from our own experience what it feels like to be ill and to suffer, it's easier to appreciate the suffering of others. It's a fact, however, that many doctors have experienced predominantly good health. If you haven't suffered a severe illness yourself, you should still try to imagine how it would feel. If you don't become sensitive to the mental and emotional experiences that patients are having, you tend to focus only the physical mechanics of being ill. Illness includes both the disease and the person's reaction to their own body. So the first step in becoming more compassionate is to learn how it feels to be ill. Once we truly understand how illness is experienced—the anguish and pain that is involved—we can more naturally respond with the wish to alleviate it. Compassion, as I mentioned above, is the wish to alleviate suffering. One of the first steps in becoming more compassionate is understanding clearly the nature of suffering.

3

What Patients Are Looking For

THE BENEFITS of cultivating a compassionate attitude become more clear if we focus on the way that caregivers are perceived by people in pain. When a person is in pain, the connection with the caregiver can affect them in powerful ways—in the way the caregiver looks, how they speak, and what they do. When the caregiver is especially kind in that situation, it makes a really big difference.

When people are ill, whether the suffering is predominantly physical or predominantly mental, where do they turn for help? They go to a medical professional. They choose a medical professional because they feel that a doctor or nurse is the person most likely to be able to help them. When patients are seriously ill, their physical situation may be amplified by a lot of anguish and fear. They develop a great deal of hope that the doctor will be able to help them, but the hope is countered by the fear that nothing can be done, that perhaps the situation is hopeless.

When such a person encounters a doctor or nurse who actually cares and can demonstrate that they care, it makes a tremendous difference. If you are a caregiver, you should try to convey reassurance to the patient, such as: "I really care about you. I'll do my best, not just in regard to diagnosis and treatment. I won't just use you to prove my medical skills. If there is something that I don't know about, I won't be afraid to ask others. There is a whole array of medical resources:

doctors, books, nurses. I'll consult all that are necessary for your benefit." If patients get the feeling that someone really cares about them and wants to help them, their fear diminishes. They feel that there is some hope, and they become much more receptive to treatment because they trust the caregiver. In this way, genuine concern and compassion make a huge difference.

Disease is one of the things we worry about the most. As a result, doctors are very important in people's lives because everyone gets sick. It's not just a theoretical concern. As a matter of fact there is no worry worse than the fear of illness and death. When someone is actually ill, someone who can remove the fear of illness, or the fear of dying, is the greatest help. It is the nicest way to help someone else.

Although medicine is a huge subject, a doctor still manages to learn, in a broad sense, most of it. Afterward that knowledge is put to use in order to assist other people. The greatest assistance can be offered when it comes to helping someone who is about to die, because they often have the most suffering. When a doctor prescribes medicine, or performs surgery, or helps take care of a dying patient in a very kind and caring fashion, the patient can feel the physician's compassion. It gives the patient a deep sense of relief. It creates a feeling deep down in the patient that helps to alleviate the patient's mental distress and pain.

From the moment someone is born there is the constant danger of falling ill or dying. This constant uncertainty, along with the fact that we actually become ill many times in our lives, confirms the importance of doctors. Sickness and dying are so common that a doctor will always have work to do. In fact, doctors may end up feeling that the burden of taking care of sick people is too much. They have to deal with so many painful situations—so many people who are in pain and dying. When people are seriously ill, their main object of hope becomes the doctor. If someone holds religious beliefs, they may pray to God, but their immediate source of hope is the doctor. This is how sick people think. Sick people may feel that a doctor is like their father or mother—someone who can save them and nurture them back to health. All of a sudden the patient feels him or herself in the role of a child. The doctor is the parent, and the patient puts trust in just one place—the doctor.

When people are sick and anxious, they become more sensitive. At that point in time they will notice acutely every little facial expression in the doctor. If there is a slight change in the doctor's demeanor, they feel it. Patients react to the doctor's body language, the movement of the facial muscles, and especially the eyes. Our eyes convey a lot of meaning. You all know what is meant by the term "loving gaze." Joy, sadness, or fear can be discerned in someone's eyes, and the sick person is able to see this more easily.

The patient has just one concern: "How do I get better? The doctor must make me better as soon as possible." Being sick is like having an acutely painful thorn stuck in your arm. You just want the doctor to pull it out as quickly as he or she can. That's the patient's attitude.

What the patient is really trying to determine is whether the doctor is putting his or her full attention toward the patient's problem. The patient feels that the problem can be fixed if the doctor just pays enough attention. The patient has the attitude: "If the doctor gives his or her full attention to my problem, they can fix it." That's how it appears from the patient's point of view. If they sense that the doctor has not put their mind fully on their problem, they remain fearful.

The doctor views the patient in the context of his or her medical training. The doctor has learned how to make a diagnosis and how to apply treatment. During his or her training, the doctor has been taught how to behave toward a patient, how to control their facial reactions, how to modulate their way of speaking. However, when the doctor walks into a room with a patient, the doctor's true attitude toward the patient will be immediately visible, regardless of the attitude that the doctor attempts to portray. Something intangible is revealed that reflects the doctor's actual motivation or attitude. The caring motivation needs to be genuine, because it is perceived by the patient. It can't be faked.

In short, actually caring and wanting to help, rather than merely thinking of the patient as a problem to solve, has a tremendous effect on the patient. Fortunately, it is possible to train in these qualities, to consciously form our attitude in a positive, benevolent way. Thinking about how caregivers are perceived by those they care for is a form of wisdom, which can then be a stimulus to cultivating a compassionate attitude. In this way, we can see that we need to combine wisdom and compassion in order to most fully care for those whose suffering we would like to relieve.

4

Combining Wisdom and Compassion

WHEN IT COMES to the healing professions, wisdom means knowing what it takes, understanding all the factors that are necessary in the healing process. It is not limited to making the correct diagnosis and applying the proper medication or surgical procedure. Wisdom incorporates the attitude of caring along with all of one's training, experience, and knowledge of disease. It is the combination of all of these factors that we can call wisdom.

Practicing the art of healing clearly involves a great deal of wisdom. What I am calling "wisdom" could also be called "intelligence," whichever you prefer. Intelligently caring for patients means finding the right solution to their problem. Not only finding a cure, but finding it quickly, and choosing the treatment that is most effective in the long run. If you happen to know the answer already, that's fine. However, if you don't know, then finding the right answer requires skill and wisdom. A wise caregiver doesn't hesitate to consult others. This willingness to consult others, and knowing when to do so, is part of what it means to have wisdom.

Other factors fall under the topic of wisdom as well, especially tolerance and perseverance on the part of the healing professional. Tolerance is incredibly important because dealing with sick people is not necessarily pleasant. They can be downright annoying. Sick people

don't take it personally

often lose their good manners. This is not something they consciously choose to do, they simply can't help it. Whether it is the fear or the pain, or the drugs they are taking, patients can get intoxicated and lose their manners. They may insult you, not because they want to, but because they can't help it. One sign of wisdom on the healing professional's part is not taking this personally, thinking instead, "Oh, he's disturbed, he can't help it. He's usually a gentleman, but today, unfortunately, he doesn't behave like one. I don't need to take it personally. He's just not in control right now." Some kind of tolerance is always necessary, but especially when caring for sick people.

As I mentioned above, the patient may relate to the doctor like a father or mother, and begin acting like a child. When children are happy they hug other family members. When they are unhappy, they cry, and may even physically strike family members. It's precisely those moments we need to have tolerance and patience. That's when we need compassion and loving-kindness. If we can maintain an attitude of compassion at those difficult times, it provides the best opportunity for healing to take place.

If we really want to be more compassionate, we need to know when compassion can make the most difference. Otherwise, we may feel most compassionate only when taking care of patients who are kind to us and appreciate our help. When faced with difficult patients, we might think, "I'm doing my best, why are they treating me like this? This man or woman is ordinarily gentle and considerate. What happened today? I'm trying my best, but they are blaming me for their discomfort." These kinds of thoughts can make you tired and unhappy—even disappointed and angry. At that point, the practice of medicine begins to feel burdensome. You might even consider giving up, thinking, "I can't deal with this anymore." You feel like you're not doing a good job, that somehow you should have done better. Your sense of duty tells you to carry on, but you begin to think that you can't take it anymore. There is a tug-of-war on your emotions. That tug-of-war robs you of your enthusiasm, disturbs others, and prevents you from doing your job smoothly. It even interferes with your ability to make good decisions. You lose your sense of wisdom, patience, and tolerance. You can begin to be disturbed in other aspects of your life as well.

With wisdom, we can see how this process works. Without wisdom, we may know that we should be more compassionate, but we just can't figure out how to do it, and we end up feeling discouraged. Again, we need to understand that illness is not only physical—physical illness can lead to mental unbalance. We need to remember that the patient is unable to control what they say because they are too scared, too panicked, and in too much pain. If we have insight into the cause of their behavior, we can take it less seriously, less personally. It won't become such a burden to us or make us discouraged. If we know the reason behind the patient's actions and emotions, we become more tolerant, which allows us to be more compassionate. At the same time, we begin to feel more satisfaction, and our hearts feel lighter. We think, "Even though I'm confronting these difficult problems, I'm actually doing well." We can rejoice in ourselves.

From one perspective, we could say that all of this stems from the power of loving-kindness. For example, when a child has a problem, the mother has enough endurance to care for that child twenty-four hours a day. She will do whatever is necessary. If the child cannot sleep, the mother does not need to sleep. Of course her body gets tired, and mentally she gets fatigued, but she is very motivated to care for her dear child. Tolerance and patience are already present. The mother does not need to consciously work to build up the necessary patience or tolerance. All of these qualities arise naturally due to the loving-kindness of the mother. If your loving-kindness declines, then your patience and tolerance decline automatically. If you have no loving-kindness at all, then your diligence, tolerance, and interest in doing your work will all fall to zero.

In summary, the healing professional should not only deal with the patient's body, but needs to understand what it feels like to be sick. You need to comprehend how painful, how worrisome, and how disturbing it can be to not know what is going to happen to yourself. Understanding the interplay of all these factors requires wisdom. A true understanding of how these factors impact the behavior of a specific patient is what allows compassion to grow.

5

Impermanence, the Body, and the Senses

I F WE COMPARE humans to animals and all other forms of sentient beings, the human body has a much greater capacity to influence others. As I've already mentioned, when a human sets out to do good, it is possible to do so on a great scale. On the other hand, a person who sets out to do evil can also carry that out on a tremendous scale. Therefore, while we have the most capable of life forms, wouldn't it be better to direct ourselves to do what is good and meaningful?

If we choose to orient ourselves toward doing something beneficial and noble, we should begin right away, because the amount of time we have left in our lives is uncertain. Life does not go on forever. This lifetime is not permanent. As soon as we are born, we draw closer to our own death with every passing moment. This sad fact is actually one of the hardest things to contemplate. And it's not just death that we can't avoid. We also cannot prevent aging, and we cannot really prevent falling ill. When we are ill, we are unable to carry out noble deeds, and when we get old, we are not able to function as well as when we were younger. This is why we need to pursue noble activity at this time, while we still have the chance.

Everything that is formed is impermanent. We need to recognize the reality of that statement for ourselves. Up until now there has not been anything in this world that after having been formed did not fall apart or perish. There haven't been any things or beings that have not fallen apart or died in the past, and we can safely apply this observation to the future as well. That is what is meant by the Buddhist saying, "All formed things perish, they are impermanent." We can understand this. It's obvious when we think about it. We need to understand that every birth ends in death. Death is certain, but the circumstances and the time are not fixed.

Likewise, everything we perceive, all the things surrounding us, change constantly, including our relationship with others. An inescapable fact of impermanence is that every meeting ends in separation. We will eventually be separated from whomever we meet or know in our lives. We may separate from them temporarily many times, and we will eventually have a final separation. Whether we are friends, enemies, relatives, or lovers, we all separate. This is just the nature of things. If it happens that we don't want to separate, then it's painful. If someone is so dear to you that you feel you could never stand to be apart from them, there's still nothing you can do to prevent it. The pain can be unbearable.

The same holds true for everything that one accumulates or builds. If we inspect matter closely, we find that it changes every instant. Everything gets used up or scattered in the end. Buildings crumble and fall apart. There is no exception. This is what Buddhism refers to as the "impermanence of all things."

Suffering has a lot to do with impermanence. Because things are impermanent, there is suffering. Not wanting to age, we still age. It's painful. We don't want to be ill, but no one can completely prevent illness. Even doctors get sick. No one wants to die, but they still do. Why does it happen this way? Because everything is impermanent. Otherwise everything would remain the same, without changing. If you were in good health, you would stay in good health continuously. If things were not impermanent, you would not get older, you would not have to look forward to losing your good health. But it doesn't happen that way. Thus, impermanence is the cause of a lot of pain.

We often think of happiness as the opposite of suffering. We should investigate what we mean by "happiness." Does happiness have a location? Is it something outside ourselves? Is it inside ourselves? Somewhere in between? The normal tendency is to feel that happiness is over there, at some distance from us, and not in our direct control. So we think that until we get to that other place—until we get within reach of happiness—we will remain unhappy. If we try to measure happiness, it's hard to put a finger on it. What would perfect happiness feel like? Can it be achieved by surrounding ourselves with pleasurable objects and friends? Would that be true happiness or not?

My opinion is that whenever there is a moment of being content, whenever there is a moment of feeling, "this is all right," that is a moment of happiness. The person who never experiences a moment of contentment—who is never satisfied—is never happy. They couldn't possibly be. When someone lacks basic necessities, such as food or shelter, that is a cause of pain and suffering. But someone who has everything also suffers. That may seem strange. It's easy to understand why people who are destitute and lack the necessities of life could suffer. But someone who possesses the usual descriptions of pleasure and luxury, that they should have reasons to suffer doesn't seem right. In fact, it's sometimes true that a rich person might suffer more than a poor person, because it's harder for a rich person to be content. One root of suffering is discontent; not knowing how to be content prevents happiness.

If we examine the human body, we can see that it is a combination of many components, such as flesh, blood, bones, sinews, and marrow. As long as there is some breathing and warmth, the body continues to live, and we call that "the living human body." The physical body is a container for a lot of different things. There is the skin that covers it, and then there are the components that are found inside. Ironically, many of the things humans consider to be the most disgusting and repulsive are actually found within the living human body. If we don't think about what is inside, we can look at another person's form and perhaps feel quite attracted to them. The face is lovely, the skin is smooth, and various features may be extremely enticing. But as many of you know, if you cut into a human body, a lot of things get revealed that most people don't see on a daily basis. There's blood, lymph, muscles, fat, urine, and half-digested or fully digested food that is destined to become excrement. All of that is exposed when you cut open a body. And suddenly it's not that attractive.

Yet this is what we live with, this is what we walk around with. Now when this combination of components—which is what the human body is—becomes ill, either through an external disturbance or an imbalance in the internal elements, the result is something that is experienced as "dis-ease." Suddenly, we are not well. Then we ask, "Why did this happen?" According to the Buddhist tradition, there are two reasons for disease. One is called past karma, meaning the ripening of cause and effect from the past, and the other is called temporary circumstance. Now when something is the ripening of past karma, there is not always the possibility for a cure. Past karma can be the explanation for the fact that some people fall ill more than others, and some people, for no obvious reason, have a lot of unhappiness, depression, and other forms of mental disease. Karma can also lead to physical disease. Sometimes these conditions are curable and sometimes they are not. Besides karmic causes, there are also diseases due to temporary circumstances, for which there is also sometimes a cure, and sometimes not.

The body is such a precarious, fragile system that it doesn't take much to put it out of balance so that it no longer feels well. In the Buddhist tradition, the body is occasionally referred to as "the heap that is the repository for pain and suffering." The body is always just ready to fall ill. Perhaps the environment is a little too cold or a little too hot. Your skin is so sensitive that you may feel sudden intense discomfort the moment a mosquito bites or a bee stings. The body has a readiness to not feel well. That is due to just one of the senses—the sense of touch. But the other senses are also primed to feel discomfort.

The sensory impressions that are presented to our minds have an immediate influence on us, creating either a pleasant or an unpleasant experience. The moment you see something lovely, there's an impulse to touch it, to become involved and fascinated. If we see something a little bit desirable, we want it. If we see something a little bit awful, we are repelled. Or we may see something about which we are indifferent, and feel dull or bored. If we are experiencing things mainly with our eye sense, we can usually deal with it. But we also perceive in other ways. Suppose you are at a concert by a string quartet when a fire alarm accidentally goes off, making a terrible clanging noise. You would be both startled and irritated. We can also be disturbed by noxious smells, bad tastes, or substances that feel disgusting to our sense of touch. Even when we are relaxed and our thoughts are wandering here and there, we may think of something good, or something bad, and experience emotional responses just to our own thoughts.

There's a saying in Buddhist philosophy: "Appearances are beguiling and the mind is fickle." When appearances—meaning what is presented through the senses—are especially beguiling, we tend to get overstimulated. Our lack of stability causes our minds to immediately react to whatever is happening, either by desiring or rejecting. It is such a pervasive preoccupation that when we look back on our lives it can seem as if we spent all our time either chasing or running away from things. We pursue relationships with people and objects as if they were lasting and permanent, and then are disappointed when they are not.

The five senses tend to fool the mind. If we remain susceptible to constantly being tricked and tempted by our senses, we cannot claim to be in charge of our lives. We cannot truly say that we are independent or free. I mentioned earlier that our basic nature is compassionate and wise. If that's true, then why don't compassion and wisdom arise automatically? Why do we need to train our compassion and wisdom if they are already our basic nature?

The answer is that we are unable to simply experience our basic nature due to the ingrained tendency we have to get caught up and preoccupied by our sensory experiences and our thoughts. We allow our senses to control us, and that prevents us from being natural and free. We need to learn to perceive things as they really are. The main obstacle that prevents us from simply resting in a state of natural mind is the tendency we have to cling to the existence of ourselves as observers that are separate from the things that we observe. This tendency is called *dualistic thinking*. As long as we engage in dualistic thinking we cannot experience 100 percent peace. We can't experience being completely and naturally at ease.

Understanding what is meant by dualistic thinking is difficult, but it is the core of the Buddhist insight into reality. I will explain this in more detail below.

6

Dualistic Thinking
and Why It Is Important

WE'VE ALREADY SEEN that our constant need to react to our sensory impressions keeps us from feeling completely open and at ease. Our natural state of mind, on the other hand, is able to perceive, but it does not form concepts about what is perceived. It is from within this state of empty *open* awareness that our natural compassion and wisdom grows forth. Not forming concepts about what we perceive means learning to recognize that all that we experience is simply the play of our own mind.

Duality refers to a separation of our perception into some feeling of "self" and some feeling of "other"—a sense of a perceiver and something to be perceived. These two concepts, subject and object, form a duality, in that neither can be seen to exist without the other. Holding these two thoughts together—a separate subject and a separate object—is what is referred to by the term "clinging to duality." Although the idea of an observer and something to be observed seems to describe a completely logical way of viewing the world, clinging to duality is actually just a choice that we make—albeit an unconscious choice. However, this way of perceiving leads to consequences.

The person who feels that something is being experienced is called "me" or "I." The concept of "me" or "I" creates some fondness for ourselves, a subtle form of attachment. At the same time, it engenders a slight distancing of ourselves from those objects that are perceived as being "other than me," and this is a very subtle form of aversion. As long as we hold these concepts of separation in our mind—subject here, object there—we are prevented from knowing our true nature. Recognizing our true nature means knowing that there is no real basis for this dualistic way of perceiving. Dualistic perception is dissolved in any moment in which we are able to experience empty awareness. The lack of knowing our true nature is called *ignorance*. Therefore, at any given moment in which duality is held in mind, all three basic negative emotions—attachment, aversion, and ignorance—are present on a subtle level.

Like and dislike are emotions that we are all familiar with. In their more intense forms, we know them as attachment and anger. Where do they come from? What is their real source? Perhaps this sounds like a strange question. Some people are motivated to find out, but a lot of people have never thought about it. We are all aware that suffering exists—the experience of pain is hard to ignore. Everyone feels pain whether they comprehend its cause or not. If we could understand the true causes of suffering, we might be able to help alleviate or prevent suffering in ourselves and others. One possible answer is that the seeds of suffering are actually present in the emotions that flow from dualistic thinking. This is the Buddhist explanation. Let's look at it more closely.

Whatever we do, whether good or harmful, plants a seed that can ripen in the future. The deeds that we do are called *karmic actions*. But what leads to good or harmful actions? Whenever duality is held in mind, selfish emotions arise, and these in turn drive our behavior—our thoughts, words, and deeds. On a more subtle level, karmic actions are generated whenever *any* concept, selfish or virtuous, is held in mind. The forming of thoughts that hold things as having a separate existence from our mind is the most subtle basis for all our feelings and actions. The thought that separates the perceiver from the objects or people that are being perceived becomes the basis for subsequent emotions or actions related to that object or person. If we didn't perceive something as being separate from our own awareness, we would not be able to generate a negative emotion or action toward that object.

This process of clinging to duality is often broken down into three concepts: that there is a perceiver, that there is something to be perceived, and that there is an act of perceiving. When we look at something, such as a flower, in that first instant we are already generating concepts. "There is a flower" is one concept. "I perceive the flower" is another concept. "Noticing that we are seeing the flower" is the third concept.

Simply forming the concepts of subject, object, and action is sufficient for creating karma. *Karma* means action, and all actions have consequences or results, even this very subtle conceptuality. As long as our mind forms concepts, karma will be generated. Something is said to be created at the moment that the concept of a perceiver, that which is perceived, and the action between them is formed. That something is called a karmic action.

Karma is a Sanskrit word. Karma is also a Buddhist belief. But there is a similar concept in Western thinking. In the West we have the terms "good luck" and "bad luck." Right now we are discussing the question of *why* there is suffering. Where does suffering come from? Is it just due to bad luck? If things are going well, is that due to good luck? Why do some people have good luck, and why do some people have bad luck? Some people don't look for a reason, they simply believe that both good fortune and bad fortune are due to accident or chance—to luck.

Buddhist teachings state that good and bad fortune have a cause. They don't occur by accident or by chance. However, whether something happens to you due to a specific cause or due to chance, it still feels the same. There's no separate explanation in Buddhism about how suffering should feel—it feels the same for everyone, all over the world. What we are discussing are the possible explanations for the *cause* of suffering. To understand the cause of suffering, we need to understand selfish emotions, and what causes selfish emotions.

When the claim is made that karma is the cause of suffering, there is often some resistance. It's not part of the Western worldview, and people often find it difficult to accept. Karma begins with the forming of a concept, the forming of an attitude or opinion about something. That is how karma is made. All of the negative emotions that are generated through the forming of concepts lead to consequences in the future. Only when we rest in our own intrinsic wakefulness, in the natural mind, is the formation of karma interrupted.

Most people would like to be free of attachment and anger, because those emotions create suffering. But in order to be free from attachment and anger, we first need to know what causes those emotions. Clinging to duality creates the platform from which we react to objects and people with either attachment or anger. In the absence of the dualistic perspective, there is no way to generate a negative emotion, and thus no way to create karma that causes future suffering. This is the connection between the mental state we call duality and the causes of suffering. If anger and attachment are the cause of suffering, then eliminating dualistic thinking will eliminate future suffering. If we wish to be free from suffering, we need to address the root cause. Otherwise, we end up with a situation of trying be free of negative emotions without eliminating what caused them in the first place. It can't happen.

There are many ways in which we experience suffering. As I mentioned, human beings suffer when they are born, while they age, when they are sick, and when they die. But there are additional kinds of pain a human being experiences. One is to be unfulfilled. That in itself is painful. We want something, but it's not happening. The different variations of our yearnings are endless. In addition to not getting what we want, unwanted things happen to us again and again. Life doesn't turn out as we would like. To put it succinctly, the basis for all of this suffering is hope and fear. Each moment of our thoughts is suffused with the hope that something we want will come to pass, and the fear that something we don't want will also happen. If every moment of thought carries either hope or fear, it is extremely difficult to be 100 percent at ease, to have 100 percent peace and freedom from suffering.

Hope stems from attachment, and fear stems from aversion or anger. Thus, the only way to ever be completely at peace is to get beyond both hope and fear, to get beyond the dualistic clinging that allows those emotions to take root.

7
Conceptual and
Nonconceptual Compassion

I T MIGHT SEEM as if the concept of "clinging to duality" is just a unique philosophical point unrelated to the topic of compassion. However, we are not just addressing the benefits of compassion, but how we can make compassion more vast and less limited. In order to do that, we need to understand the difference between conceptual and nonconceptual compassion. In order to appreciate the vast potential represented by the concept of nonconceptual compassion, we need to understand the concept of duality.

While we would all agree that our compassion should be less limited, it is not so easy to know how to make this happen. We want to develop a quality of compassion that is not just directed toward a few people, but is ready to embrace anyone, without prejudice. Compassion is not simply an attitude that we can put on, like a mask, in order to present an appearance of kindness and compassion toward everyone we meet. There is a real difference between just acting as if we are kind and open to everyone and actually feeling kindness and compassion for all people. Fortunately, there is a way to develop kindness and compassion that is genuine. Moreover, once it is developed, genuine compassion is less taxing than contrived compassion. There is a Buddhist saying that "open-minded intelligence allows for boundless compassion." Once we have experienced what is truly meant by open-minded intelligence, compassion follows naturally. We can learn to train in open-minded intelligence, but it requires the understanding of some subtle concepts. Learning to fully understand just this one phrase could take months or even years.

There are two approaches to training in open-minded intelligence suffused with compassion. The first method requires conscious effort. We use our intellect to generate a distinct wish to be more compassionate, and then we steer our mind toward a compassionate attitude that embraces everyone. This method is called training in conceptual compassion. The other method is to just let it happen naturally, without premeditation. We simply let go of any concepts about how things should be, and allow ourselves to exist in a way that is totally open and compassionate. This method is called training in nonconceptual compassion. Although it sounds like it would be the easier path, nonconceptual compassion can't be experienced without using some method or training. It doesn't happen spontaneously. Although we need to make a conscious effort in order to train, the goal is to eventually experience compassion as something natural and open, not requiring conscious effort.

When our compassion derives from a deliberate effort, we may find it is easy to be compassionate toward certain people. For example, it feels natural to be kind to people that we already know and like and who appreciate us. In other situations, however, our compassion becomes more selective. Depending on our mood, we may be kind to some people but not to others. And on rarer occasions, stress in our lives may render us capable only of extremely limited compassion, unable or unwilling to help all but a few people. When our compassion depends on a conscious effort, it may not be stable.

This deliberate type of compassion is familiar to us. We call it conceptual compassion—we think of a specific person in a specific situation and we cultivate a feeling of kindness and compassion toward them. We may or may not have put much effort into training to be that way, but at least that type of compassion is familiar to us.

This deliberate type of compassion is in contrast to a more natural compassion that is free of any concepts, what I referred to above as nonconceptual compassion. As I mentioned, nonconceptual compassion comes about through open-minded intelligence. Nonconceptual compassion naturally arises from a particular state of mind called *thought-free wakefulness*. Thought-free wakefulness is a way of being that is aware and yet holds no particular thought in mind. The compassion and affection that spontaneously springs out of this state of mind is limitless. It is not confined to any particular person or situation. However, unless we are able to personally experience that state of mind, the spontaneous arising of such compassion may seem incomprehensible, or at least unattainable.

The compassion and loving-kindness that we associate with buddhas and bodhisattvas arises out of thought-free wakefulness. When I use the words buddha or buddhas you may be thinking of just one particular teacher who lived in Nepal and India long ago. I should explain a little bit about what that word actually means. The word *buddha* literally means "purified and perfected." It refers to a state of purity and perfection that is naturally present after something has been cleared away or gotten rid of. Any sentient being can attain the state of purity and perfection that is defined by the word *buddha,* and countless beings have done so. The historical Buddha is just one example.

The mental constructs that prevent us from recognizing our basic nature are called obscurations. There are two types of obscurations. The first type is referred to as *negative emotions,* of which there are ultimately 84,000 different types. We won't list them all, but the three primary ones, which I noted above, are attachment, aversion, and ignorance. There are also a few others of significance, such as jealousy and pride. These negative emotions are sometimes called *mental poisons.*

They can be thought of as shortcomings in our human nature, in our minds, and they are considered negative because they lead to suffering.

The second type of obscuration is called the *cognitive obscuration*. Compared to the negative emotions, which are easier to recognize, the second form of obscuration is much more difficult to identify and thus more difficult to be free of. Cognitive obscuration refers to our habit of clinging to duality.

Cognitive obscuration describes the tendency of our mind to cling to the threefold concepts: perceiver, that which is perceived, and the action between them. Whenever these threefold concepts arise in our mind, then this forms the basis for negative or selfish emotions to be created. As long as this tendency to form the threefold concepts is not brought to an end, then our selfish emotions do not end. Certainly this is not easy to understand conceptually and even harder to put into practice. However, the buddhas and the bodhisattvas have completely purified both types of obscurations. They have attained a purity of mind that is an inspiring example for the rest of us.

When the buddhas are said to be purified and perfected, it means that the negative emotions and the cognitive obscuration are no longer present in their minds. This purified state provides room for an incredible intelligence and compassion to manifest. The purified aspect means that the emotional obscurations and the cognitive obscurations have dissolved. What is "perfected" is profound intelligence and compassion that are not dependent on our transient thoughts and emotions.* The basis of training in nonconceptual compassion is to

---

* One of the most basic insights of Buddhist philosophy is that our mind has an awareness that is not based on thoughts and emotions. This state is referred to as *emptiness,* but rather than being a true void, this empty awareness beyond thoughts has inherent qualities. These inherent qualities are compassion and wisdom, which, when they spring from this empty nature, are felt to be more vast than the compassion and intelligence that comes from our conscious thoughts.

recognize our basic nature, purified of the two obscurations. In other words, to go beyond dualistic thinking to a state of mind that can make room for our inherent compassion and intelligence to manifest without limitation. The training involves learning to observe our thoughts and to relax our minds in a profound way. The next section of the book will focus on how one can actually begin to train in nonconceptual compassion.

TRAINING

8

What Does It Mean to Be a Spiritual Practitioner?

WHAT SETS A SPIRITUAL PRACTITIONER apart from an ordinary person? The main difference is that when a thought forms in the mind of a spiritual practitioner, the degree of clinging to things as being solid, real, and permanent is not as strong. The spiritual practitioner is striving to see things as they really are, not as they seem. This is a crucial point. When you begin to loosen the grip that makes you view everything as being solid and permanent, you are starting on the path that can allow you to decrease the effect of negative emotions and cognitive obscurations and to allow your natural good qualities to unfold. Such a person then deserves the name "spiritual practitioner."

It is not a simple task to change the way we view reality. The process is made more difficult by a particular trait that marks our present time: people want immediate gratification—instant results. Achieving a relaxed and peaceful mind, however, is not as easy as pressing a button on a machine that we could buy. If it were, we would just buy the machine, press the button, and then immediately feel relaxed, and we would be done with that. Unfortunately, our minds are not so simple. I will use this chapter to show how we can begin to change the way we view reality.

Reality is not solid and permanent. The true nature of reality can be appreciated when we are resting "free of thoughts, yet vividly perceiving." This is different from our usual perspective, in which we believe that if we don't have thoughts or concepts about an experience, then there is no way to process that information. We need to get beyond the fear that "no thoughts" means that we would be unable to function. This fear is ungrounded.

A lot of people have tried to describe what our minds are really like—philosophers, scientists, and spiritual seekers. It is difficult to define exactly what we mean by the term *mind*. One thing I think we can all agree upon is that our minds are capable of having experiences. We can describe mind as "invisible and yet powerful." We call the mind invisible because we cannot see it with our eyes, hear it with our ears, or hold it in our hands. That's what invisible means. Yet, it is powerful because of the ability to produce either good or evil.

The Buddha describes mind as "empty cognizance," meaning that the nature of mind of any sentient being is an emptiness that is at the same time awake and aware. What does *empty* mean in this context? Something with no form, shape, or color is appropriately described by the word empty. For instance, empty can describe the air or space in front of us. Because the space around us has no form, shape, or color, we could call it *empty space*. We might ask whether there is in fact such a thing as space, or whether it is more appropriate to say space does not exist. If you admit that there is such a thing as space, can you point to it? Yes or no? If you can't point to it, does that mean that space does not exist? Given the choice of saying whether there is such a thing as space or not, we have to say that there is space. There is no way around it.

If you answer that space does not exist because we can't see it, then how would you know if a door is open or closed? If you couldn't see space on the other side of a doorway, you couldn't be confident about walking through it. Yet when you look through the doorway, you do see that there is space on the other side. Since that is the case, you have to admit that you can see space, that space exists. Therefore, we can agree that we can see space.

There are actually two meanings when we use the word *see*. We can say that we "see" because there is, in fact, some object that we see. But when there is nothing present, we can also say that we "see" that there is nothing there. We are often reluctant to use the words "I see" when there is no object to be seen. The usual meaning of the word *see* more often refers to the act of observing an object. We feel that if we can't see a particular object, we shouldn't say "see."

But through my example, we can agree that *see* also refers to observing that there is in fact nothing to be seen. One can say, "I see that there is nothing there." Even if space cannot be seen, the fact that there is nothing to see is also a valid experience. We *experience* space by moving through it. We know that empty space exists. Why? When a door is open, we know there is some open space on the other side. It is not solid. We perceive the open space and feel confident that we can move through the doorway into that open area without hitting our bodies against anything. We have confidence based on our past experience—we have done it before. The reason I'm saying this is because it means that it is possible to "see" that there is nothing to see. We can have the experience of confirming that there is nothing there. We do this every day. We know that space exists, even though we can't see it or grasp it.

When the Buddha said that the mind is empty cognizance, he meant that there is no real "thing" to be seen or grasped that we can label as "mind," yet at the same time, the mind is capable of experiencing—it exists. This empty quality of our mind is not something we have to develop. Mind is already empty, naturally and originally. We do not need to make it that way. At the same time, even though mind is naturally empty, without solidity, it is able to experience or perceive whatever takes place, in a very free and open way. That is what we call *cognizance*.

When the cognizant quality of our minds clings and holds on to whatever it experiences, that clinging becomes the basis for selfish emotions to take over, as we noted in the last chapter. However, when the cognizant quality of this mind clings to nothing at all, but just openly experiences, that is called *original wakefulness*. It can also be called *all-knowing wisdom*.

Mind is empty and yet cognizant. If this empty cognizance is allowed to not cling at all, that is called the awakened state of a buddha. That is a state in which there is no forming of karma based on confusion and selfish emotions. However, at the very moment the cognizant quality clings and holds on to any concept, in the same moment there is a forming of confused, selfish emotions and karmic action.

So how do we come to experience compassion that holds no bounds? And how do we develop intelligence and awareness that is totally open and free from prejudice? Both the intelligence and the compassion come directly from our empty cognizance when it does not cling. This is not something that can be fully understood by just hearing about it; it needs to be experienced. How can we come to have this type of experience? We begin by allowing ourselves to be at ease and relaxed. The more open and relaxed we can be, the more compassionate, the more intelligent we will become. We can train in being open and relaxed, and we will discuss this in the ensuing chapters of this section.

There are two aspects of fully developed intelligence, or the intelligence of a buddha. One is to clearly see the nature of things exactly as they are. The other is to clearly and distinctly perceive all that exists. In Buddhist philosophy, these two aspects of intelligence are called "the knowledge of the unconditioned nature of things seen as they are," and "the knowledge of the conditioned perceiving of things whatever possibly exists." These definitions may may sound strange to most people. It might help to explain a bit more.

Of the two aspects of intelligence—knowing the nature of things, and perceiving all things—science is mostly concerned with the latter. When we investigate our environment scientifically, we feel that the facts of reality are self-evident—they exist in the way they appear to us. The Buddha also taught about reality, but as he did so he focused on both kinds of intelligence. What if we were to investigate time and matter? When we don't question or investigate very closely, it seems as if time and matter actually exist. But if we look closely we fail to find anything that is actually "time" or "matter" anywhere.

Let's take a simple example. Right now you are probably sitting in what we call a room. Now try pointing at "the room" with your finger. Whatever is in the direction that is indicated by your pointing finger, that by itself cannot be considered "the room." Correct? The ceiling is not "the room," the floor is not "the room," the wall is not "the room," the window is not "the room," and the door is not "the room." Whatever items the room is made of are also, individually, not the room. Wallpaper is not "the room," bricks are not "the room," wood is not "the room." But when all these different building materials are put on top of one another and arranged in a particular way, we form a concept that we are in something called a "room." We then believe that this thought is true—that there is actually something that has an inherent separate existence called "room."

We can apply the same kind of analysis to the perceiver as well. Who is it that is perceiving this room, or reading this book? The person reading this book is called a human being. What is it that we actually mean by the term human being? We could say a human being is made up of a body, a voice, and a knower, what we call mind. That sounds correct, doesn't it? But what is a human body really? And where is it? As long we don't investigate too closely, it's quite easy to give an answer. We have no doubt. From the top of the head to the soles of the feet, that is what we call "the body." We all know this. But if we choose to define the body in this way, it's pretty unsophisticated. If we are very precise about it, it is difficult to define and pinpoint the human body.

Focus for a moment on the upper part of the body from the top down to the neck. That itself is not "the body." It has a different label than "body." It's called "head." Then we have parts called "chest," "belly," "legs," "hands," and "arms." Each of these, if you took them off and put them elsewhere, would not be considered, by themselves, "the body." However, if we put all the pieces back together again, people would then say, "Oh, a body." This is pretty strange.

Similarly, each of us has a face. On the one hand, faces are pretty similar. Everybody has one nose. There are no people with two noses, I don't think. We all have two eyes, not three eyes. From that perspective we are pretty similar. The definition of the word *face* is not the same as the head, and it's not same as the neck. It just refers to the front side of the head. Usually the ears are not included. Just the part that faces outwardly is called "the face."

That's pretty simple. Now try pointing at your face with one finger. The finger will point to your nose. Or your cheek. Or your eye. No matter where your finger points, it is called something else. Yet, we seem to have no doubt when we look at someone that we are seeing their face. Afterward, we can say confidently, "I saw his or her face." We have no doubt that we saw someone's face. Let me create some doubt here.

We have what is called a visual capacity based on the presence of our eyes. Our vision is very capable. From where I'm sitting right now, I can see a whole mountain range. If you could see these mountains, you would think, "I see the mountains. They're beautiful. A lovely landscape." That seems straightforward, doesn't it?

However, we don't really see the whole mountain range. We can't even see one mountain at a time. In fact, we can't even see one person's face. Try and look at a person's face at this moment. It doesn't matter whether you look from a distance or if you look at someone close by. You can even look at your own face in a mirror. Now direct your full attention to the forehead. Now, while focusing on the forehead, can you see the chin at the same moment? When you are looking closely at the right cheek, can you really see the left cheek at the same instant? Can you even see the entire nose at the same time? Can we even say that we really see the entire tip of the nose at the same time? If we start to investigate in this way, it becomes questionable whether what is happening actually deserves the label "seeing." This can also be applied to the process of hearing, or tasting, or touching. Actually it's something very strange that takes place.* But as long as we don't investigate it too much, it seems as if our way of perceiving is just an everyday, normal event.

What I am trying to say is that there may be two ways to view reality. One is the perceived mode (how things seem to be), and the other is the real mode (how they actually are). The seeming and the real. In the perceived mode, no question arises about what I'm looking at. I see mountains in front of me. But in reality, truly and fundamentally, there is no real thing that is perceived, and there is no real perceiver, either. That is what is called emptiness. It's also called the nature of things.

What this means is that everything that we perceive is the result of some prior condition or confluence of circumstances. If something

---

* Chokyi Nyima Rinpoche is describing the interplay between our consciousness and our organs of perception. Although it may seem that our eyes are just a window into our brain, we actually can see only what we focus our attention on. As we narrow our attention, we find that we can see only very small pieces of the world around us at any given instant. Like a computer, our brain assembles these pieces into a coherent sense of reality. What we call reality is itself assembled from tiny bits of matter that eventually are found to have no solid basis of existence, even in modern physics. Due to the absence of solidity of matter, and our inability to see anything that we have not focused our attention on, we can no longer be certain of the phrase "Seeing is believing."

appears only as a result of some prior condition, that means that it's devoid of a true independent identity. It's empty.

This lack of independent identity can be applied to the concept of time as well. The past cannot be said to exist, because it is already in the past. The future does not exist because it has not happened yet. The present moment cannot be pinpointed either, because the moment that you define an instant of time as the present, it has already slipped into the past. "Time" exists only because we hold our experiences in mind.

What is the point of this discussion? It's an important one. If we allow any thought that forms in our consciousness to have free rein, we just get caught up in that thought involuntarily. At that moment we are not spiritual practitioners. We need to think differently. Of course thoughts will arise. But we should not experience them as an ordinary person does. We should work toward seeing things as they truly are, and not being so attached to transitory sensations and thoughts. As our involvement with passing thoughts and emotions becomes less, our inherent wisdom and compassion will begin to increase.

The Buddha taught very clearly about the origin of compassion and wisdom. The absence of thoughts and concepts allows the spontaneous expression of compassion and wisdom. It's our basic nature. The word *buddha* means "purified and perfected," and that which is perfected is compassion and wisdom. This applies not just to the Buddha, but to ourselves. We have the capacity for wisdom, and we also have the capacity for being compassionate. This is why if we train and cultivate this capacity, we can be buddhas too. This is called "the buddha appearing from within"—within ourselves—because we all have the potential for being purified and perfected. A spiritual practitioner can have no higher goal, because no higher goal exists. We become buddhas by recognizing and training a potential that is already present in all of us.

9

Developing a Compassionate Attitude

EARLIER WE MENTIONED that, among all sentient beings, humans are the most capable. This capability springs from our mind, a mind that can think. Thoughts can be virtuous or unvirtuous. Thinking in a particular way creates a habit over time. When this habit is wholesome, one is able to do tremendous good. On the other hand, if unwholesome or negative thoughts become a habit, we can end up causing harm.

For this reason, when we wake up in the morning, we should try our best to make the first thought that comes to mind a noble one—a very sincere and strong thought of doing good. We should make our first thought of the morning into a true desire to be of benefit to other beings. Then the momentum created by that positive intention can be with us for the rest of the day.

We can do even better than that. We can not only form a positive, noble attitude the moment we get up, but we can also remind ourselves of that thought every so often throughout the day. That's even more effective. Why is that? If the wholesome frame of mind that we form in the morning—that resolve—is not so strong, then it can easily be forgotten. When a thought, or a commitment to think a certain way, is strong and deeply felt, however, it does not vanish so easily. We have all experienced the fact that a deep emotion—whether positive or negative—can stay with us for the whole day and night, whether we want it to or not. If your first thought of the day is not only noble but is deeply and sincerely felt, it may permeate the atmosphere of the rest of your day.

It is also possible to exert some positive influence over our sleep state. Whenever we lay down to go to sleep, whether it is late in the evening or some other time, there is a period of time in which we are just about to fall asleep. We call it "falling asleep," but what actually happens resembles a small death. In what way is falling asleep similar to dying? The similarity is that the reality of our daytime existence subsides, and the five senses cease to function for a while. When a person falls into a deep sleep, what lies there is a breathing corpse. Waking up in the morning is similar to taking birth into this world for the first time, because the continuity of our consciousness appears to have been interrupted. Just before falling asleep, however, there's always a final thought. We can try to make that last thought a noble, benevolent thought. If we can do that, the quality of that thought can permeate our entire sleeping state. The possibility is there. We can then say, from a spiritual point of view, that our sleep has become a virtuous sleep.

Likewise, you could just doze off without any particular frame of mind—not evil, not noble, just neutral. If that happens the sleeping state will be not have any particular benefit or harm. If your last thought is selfish, or even hostile, then falling asleep with that in mind saturates the sleeping state with unwholesome emotions. This is a simple idea, but it is an important one. Without too much difficulty, without too much hardship, we can ensure that a significant portion of our lives becomes saturated with goodness. Isn't that a pleasant idea?

If you are upset and angry during the day, you can end up replaying those feelings during the night. If you feel depressed or are in pain during the day, you may experience those same feelings again in a dream. Traumatic events—something involving intense fear or shock —can also be re-experienced during the dream state. The repercussions of events in our lives can be very forceful, leading to emotional habits or patterns. Fortunately, we have the power to consciously mold our habitual tendencies. Habits of thinking are created by whatever predominates in our state of mind. So if we accustom ourselves to a noble attitude, then that can become our predominant state of mind.

If we fall asleep with a virtuous or noble frame of mind, then the odds are higher that the first thought that springs to mind when we wake up will also be virtuous or noble. That is one aspect of karma— the karmic result of consciously planting a thought in our mind. As a result of that first conscious thought, a new thought may occur that is a reflection of that first thought. It's not the same thought, but something that feels quite similar due to the power of what preceded it. That is how habits are formed. If you fall asleep feeling deeply unhappy, then the moment you wake up there will be some remnant of that feeling. It's not likely if you go to sleep feeling sad that you will wake up feeling full of joy. Isn't that true?

If we fall asleep full of joy and delight, then the odds are higher that when we wake up some of that feeling will resurface. This demonstrates something essential about the way the mind works, and we can put this knowledge to good use in our waking life. For instance, it can be very beneficial to intentionally sustain a sense of taking delight in others, and feeling kindly toward them—the emotions that we connect with having a noble frame of mind. For while that frame of mind is, of course, beneficial to others, it benefits ourselves as well. If we were to describe the benefit in economic terms, we might say we gain a sizable profit from a small investment.

We can form a compassionate, noble attitude in each and every moment, and when we do that consistently, we find that a continuity and a momentum begins to permeate our state of mind. Compassion is just a thought, a mental state. Likewise, ill will, or evil intent, is also just a state of mind. Thus, by consciously and consistently choosing compassionate thoughts, we can become more compassionate people.

We often label people as either good or unpleasant, but on what basis do we make such judgements? We might think people's personalities are intrinsically good or bad. But what we are really looking at are their mental tendencies—their habits sustained over a lifetime. In other words, we are judging whether people have accustomed themselves to noble or ignoble habitual attitudes. It is our habitual attitudes, not some core personality, that make us who we are. Therefore, it is extremely important to become accustomed to wholesome states of mind. As we grow accustomed to maintaining a noble attitude, we gradually experience the ripening of the altruistic heart, set free from any limitations or boundaries. The basis for this altruistic awakened mind is already present in all of us.

One of the first steps to becoming more compassionate, then, is to take charge of our habitual tendencies by doing three things. First, we try to change negative attitudes into neutral attitudes. Second, we try to change neutral attitudes into positive and wholesome attitudes. Finally, the wholesome frame of mind is transformed into thought-free wakefulness. Does that sound difficult? Most good things are. Acting in an unwholesome manner often seems easier to accomplish, whereas being noble can be extremely difficult. It is also difficult to make significant progress if one makes only a tiny effort. Developing a noble heart requires effort, but it is extremely meaningful. There's a huge benefit from the effort that you invest.

10

The Key to Compassion

KINDNESS AND COMPASSION are states of mind that are very clean and clear. Achieving that type of clarity and purity allows the mind to have a greater impact on others. I heard a story from the West in which a child was trapped under the weight of an automobile, and the mother was able to lift the car off the child. The mother's love for the child was so great that it imbued her body with superhuman strength for the one instant that it was needed. This is a demonstration of the power of love and affection.

Deeply felt kindness and compassion generates a clarity of mind, a sense of being present for the person you are caring for. When a doctor or nurse truly cares for a person, these feelings can produce a kind of attentiveness that makes it more difficult to make mistakes or errors in judgement. This kindness and concern also inspires confidence in the patient. The patient is able to relax, to be more at ease in a difficult situation. When the doctor has an honest and kind face and speaks words that show true concern and care, the sick person feels it a hundred times more than any other person would.

When someone who is afraid and worried encounters a capable doctor's kind words and kind face, then confidence and trust can arise. I've often heard that when the patient enjoys that kind of trust, the chances for a more rapid recovery are increased.* A number of doctors

---

* An article in *The Lancet,* one of the top medical journals in the world, drew the

have told me that if mutual trust between the surgeon and the patient has been established before a surgical procedure, the outcome is much better. This is another example of the power of kindness and compassion.

Another benefit of truly caring about your patients is that inspired thinking comes more readily; you are able to recall important information more easily. You are able to remember what you otherwise might have forgotten, and you are able to make choices that didn't seem available before. In this way compassion and kindness can actually help you function in a more intelligent manner.

When we are feeling annoyed, irritated, or even angry, we can't function as well as we would like to. At those times we are at risk of doing or saying things we otherwise wouldn't. If we are really furious, we might say words we wouldn't dream of saying in an ordinary situation. Anger can have a very strong negative power. So, while positive emotions have power, negative emotions can have power as well.

When kindness and compassion are joined with the clarity of intelligence, the combined power is truly incredible. But where do these qualities of kindness, compassion, and intelligence come from? Are they something that we already have? Definitely. A compassionate frame of mind, and the capacity for intelligence, is something that every person, animal, or any other type of being already has. It's an intrinsic quality of the mind. You can say the light of compassion is already shining, like the moon that has already risen in the sky. However, from time to time, it happens that dark clouds—of selfishness, ill will, and other negative emotions—obscure the moon. So our job

---

following conclusion from a review of studies that tried to measure the impact of compassionate care on the outcome for the patient: "One relatively consistent finding is that physicians who adopt a warm, friendly, and reassuring manner are more effective than those who keep consultations formal and do not offer reassurance." [March 10, 2001]

is to ensure that those clouds of ill will, deceit, rivalry, and so forth, are cleared from the sky. How can we do that?

We need to train ourselves in being that way. The training doesn't have to be Buddhist. Since compassion is basic to our nature, training in compassion involves removing the clouds—the obscurations— that prevent our natural compassion from shining forth. The most basic step in this regard is to learn to relax. Whatever advice or system that helps you learn to deeply relax your mind will be beneficial. Whether we follow a spiritual path, or whether we practice a religion—any type of religion—if we simply relax from deep within, we will not contradict any spiritual system. It's not possible. That's the first step.

How do we relax our minds? Any method or technique that works is fine. The best methods, however, are natural ones. There are drugs that are supposed to relax one's state of mind, and they probably work to some extent. But wouldn't it be more practical if the mind could relax itself, without being dependent on some external substance? I think we would agree that if the mind can relax itself, that is better and more beneficial. So, how do we do that?

We need to try to be at ease physically—the more relaxed the better. But it would not be sufficient to be relaxed physically and still feel mentally tense or upset. It's more important to be relaxed mentally. In fact, when we are thoroughly relaxed mentally, the body will automatically relax as well. So how do we begin to relax our mind? As long as we remain preoccupied with the endless flow of our thoughts, the mind does not relax. The more that the busyness of being caught up with our thoughts is allowed to subside, to the same extent the mind eases off and relaxes.

It is common to alternate stretches of work with periods of vacation. We can take the same approach to incorporating training within our daily activities. We can take a brief vacation from our regular activities, and we can call this break the training session. During a vacation we don't have to worry about a thing—we can forget our daily duties and responsibilities. In the same way, when we do a training session, it's a break during which we can let go of our preoccupation with thoughts. Let's say that on a daily basis we take a fifteen-minute break during which we allow ourselves, both physically and mentally, to just be at ease. That type of break creates an effect that can extend throughout the rest of the day. Its effect can allow us to reconnect with this feeling of ease amid many different situations.

Why do I call this break a training session? What are we training in? We're training our minds to not be anxious about anything, to let go of hope and fear about whatever is going on in our lives. We are also training to be nonjudgmental, to forgo judgments about what we like and what we don't like. When we develop an attraction to something or someone, we often become obsessed by that attraction. If we give ourselves over to to that attraction wholeheartedly, the pursuit creates intense stress, especially if we are not successful in attaining our desired object. The same holds true when we dislike something. The activity of trying to avoid someone or something we perceive as unpleasant also causes us distress.

What happens if we drop that approach? What if we stop mentally chasing after what we like and avoiding what we don't like? What if we just allow ourselves to mentally relax? Having a neutral frame of mind in itself can lead to a feeling of peace. One way to experience neutral feelings or thoughts is by simply noticing our own breathing. Noticing the flow of our own breath is not an especially attractive activity, and it's not repulsive, either. Also you need not fabricate something that is not already present—you are already breathing. Therefore, by using the breath to train in relaxation, we can occupy ourselves with simply noticing what is already happening. We inhale—it's happening. Then we exhale—that's also happening. We are simply paying attention in this way to something that is neutral. Automatically we feel more at ease, more relaxed. When we are relaxed and at ease with ourselves, it is much easier to spontaneously feel kind and compassionate. There's a connection between feeling relaxed and feeling compassionate. Conversely, when we feel rigid and uptight, it is much more difficult to feel compassion and kindness.

We've seen that attachment and anger are negative emotions that can disturb our mental state. In order to be deeply relaxed, we need to be unoccupied by feelings of attachment and anger, which are more blatant emotions, and also free from like and dislike, which are the same emotions on a more subtle level. Obsession and fury are an extreme escalation of attachment and aversion. If we can manage to at least be free of obsession and fury, we will of course feel more relaxed and at ease. But even if we are experiencing just a subtle form of like and dislike in our mind, this keeps us from feeling completely relaxed. Therefore, it is important to pursue a sense of complete equanimity. Equanimity means being undisturbed by like and dislike.

When we are relaxed there is a pleasant feeling—it simply feels good to be relaxed and at ease. It is also possible that being at ease mentally could reduce illness. You might get sick less often. As you know, some diseases occur when there is an imbalance between one's body and the environment. Some illnesses are due to an imbalance of different factors within the body. If the environment is too extreme, it can make you ill, and a lack of proper nutrition can lead to disease. However, some kinds of illness are produced purely through one's mental state, like harboring too much despair and grief, having too much anger and hate, and nurturing an intense jealousy. These strong emotions may make you physically sick.

Any kind of extreme emotion that is harbored too long in your mind could lead to illness. So there are many reasons why a relaxed frame of mind can be very beneficial. If you are concerned with being of assistance to others, it is better to be relaxed. There are also some personal benefits from being relaxed—one simply feels better. So, a peaceful mind is a worthwhile goal—a peaceful, kind, and intelligent frame of mind. Or we could say, "calm mind, kind mind, clear mind." Being calm allows you to be compassionate. When our kindness and compassion is allowed to be open, unbiased, and unlimited, we can experience a greater sense of clarity, an increased mental sharpness. This brings us back to the profound Buddhist phrase I introduced earlier: *emptiness suffused with compassion*. We can now begin to appreciate its deeper meaning.

I have suggested that you could spend ten to fifteen minutes a day cultivating mental relaxation. However, what about the rest of your day, beyond those fifteen minutes? We need to find a way to remind ourselves to be relaxed and present in all situations, whatever the circumstances. For whenever we feel deeply at ease with ourselves, that is the true holiday. At that very moment! You don't need to go somewhere else to achieve that. You don't need to plan ahead of time to arrange a stretch of free days in order to try to feel that way. You can give yourself that experience at any time, anywhere—even while sitting on the toilet! It requires neither a huge effort nor great expense. It is within reach immediately. How wonderful!

A relaxed frame of mind is actually the true vacation. You notice that when you return from a really satisfying vacation, your whole mood and atmosphere has changed. If the vacation went well and you were really able to relax, your stress is gone, and when you get back, you feel much more gentle and kind. Almost transformed. Where does this come from? It's the result of successfully taking a holiday from your everyday busy thoughts.

We need to *learn* to be relaxed and at ease. Is it enough to have only a few moments of peace here and there? It would be far better if we could be relaxed continuously. How is that accomplished? Every skill we learn is simply the forming of a new habit. How do we form new habits? By training, by practicing. Those who become expert at something without any training are very rare. Everything becomes easier with practice. Therefore, being at ease with yourself is something that you can train in and will become easier with practice.

However, this won't happen if we just relate to it as a theory about how you could be more relaxed. It needs to be brought into our personal experience. When we think about training in relaxation, we may feel that we don't have an extra fifteen minutes per day to spend on this project. We may also feel some resistance in our minds, thinking, "I'm not sure I really want to do that." Such thoughts don't change the fact that a certain amount of training to be at ease and relaxed can bring great benefit. This is not something that you can appreciate just by reading about it. The full benefit cannot be imparted through words. You can only gain experience from your own training.

11
Learning to Meditate

U P UNTIL NOW I have talked only about training in relaxation. However, training in relaxation is simply another term for meditation. What do we actually mean by the term *meditation*? This word refers to a wide spectrum of practices, but from the Buddhist perspective we can condense all of them into just two types. There is meditation with effort and meditation that is effortless. The effortless training is more perfect, more effective, more pure, and is able to spontaneously overcome whatever needs to be eliminated. Therefore, it's the best.

However, effortless meditation will not be effective if we have not learned to recognize our basic nature. In the absence of resting in our basic awareness, we continually get carried away. We get annoyed, we get attached, we get dull, and we cling to this and that. We are so used to experiencing the world in terms of solid subjects and objects that we feel as if there is no other way to perceive. Even when we acknowledge the strength of our habitual tendencies, and try to be spontaneous and natural and effortless, we can't quite pull it off. Something else is required. If we have not been introduced to our basic nature and we are not used to it, then we may need to employ meditation methods that require effort in order to work our way toward the day when we are able to utilize the effortless methods.

Luckily, there are many such methods to choose from, methods that have been proven by the experience of meditators over centuries. A good method immediately helps to reduce your negative emotions and immediately helps to promote your intrinsic good qualities.

When we begin to practice meditation, it is important to start with the right motivation. We need to establish the proper attitude toward our training. We can think to ourselves, "Sure, I would like to be more calm, but my main intention is to be more compassionate, to develop more insight, more wisdom, and more caring. That is why I'm spending this time practicing meditation: not simply to benefit myself, but also so that I may be of benefit to others. I want to help others to be more clear, to be more affectionate and caring." That kind of motivation is important before practicing meditation. And forming such an attitude is in itself a positive action, a good deed.

It is exactly the same when we sit down to read a book on spiritual training. It is important to put ourselves in the right frame of mind before opening it up if we want to truly benefit from our effort. We want to bring to mind a sense of joy and appreciation for the opportunity to pursue spiritual study, which is inherently a noble pursuit. You don't want to read it as if it were any other type of book, lying back, half paying attention, half dozing off. You want to sit nicely, and make sure you have made yourself more clear-minded and appreciative. You want to take delight in reading and then think to yourself, "If there is something noble in this book, I would like to incorporate that in my life. I would like to use what I understand here to bring benefit for myself and others." In this way we can understand the profound points more clearly than if we just read it in a casual way.

In the same manner, when you sit down for a meditation session, first reflect for a moment: "All right, this is wonderful. I have managed to set aside fifteen minutes (for example) for something really positive, and I will use these fifteen minutes to improve myself. That's the purpose. Through that I would like to be able to help countless others, not just a fixed number, but completely open-ended. I would like to benefit all of them through the qualities that can become manifest through this practice." In this way, there is a sense of delight when practicing during the meditation session. You can really appreciate the opportunity to practice and train in this way.* Thus, your meditation becomes much more effective, more able to bring results.

You should sit down to meditation practice with a reason. Through your reading, study, and reflection you will begin to understand the benefits of training in relaxation, in meditation. When you fully trust in these reasons, you will be able to practice with more conviction.

We know from our own personal experience that everyone has good sides and bad sides. The good side is when we are being intelligent and compassionate and kind. These qualities are actually deeply rooted in our nature, like seeds. Without these seeds, this potential for growing our own wisdom and compassion, there would be absolutely no point in trying to develop those qualities. It wouldn't be possible because without the seeds of those qualities there is no way for them to grow and expand.

The Buddha said that all sentient beings are buddhas, but their minds are covered by temporary obscurations. When the obscurations are removed, real buddhas—purified and perfected—shine forth. Our buddha nature is like a precious gemstone that has been temporarily dropped in the mud—a priceless jewel, unrecognizable right now because it is encrusted with dirt. Its true value is not apparent. Our basic nature is the priceless jewel, and the mud is our attachment, anger, and closed-mindedness. When the temporary obstructions are

---

* We may take for granted the opportunity to read about and train in Buddhist meditation practices. These practices flourished for over 1000 years in Tibet, but were abruptly curtailed when the Chinese invaded in the 1950s. Even today, the Tibetans do not enjoy complete freedom to study and practice Buddhism within their own country.

removed, we have attained liberation. Training in meditation is the way to remove the temporary obscurations.

A key point is that unless you identify the temporary obscurations as undesirable, you will not try to remove them. Why would you work to remove something that you don't believe exists in the first place or that you don't see as a problem? This is part of the process of understanding the reasons for training in meditation. When you begin to identify the temporary obscurations as being a problem—a huge problem—you become motivated to do something about it.

If you are a healing professional who meets someone who is only mildly ill, you don't take it so seriously. That's natural. However, if you encounter someone with a really severe illness, then you don't waste any time. You immediately intervene and begin treatment. Likewise, if you recognize your own obscurations as a serious problem, you automatically develop the motivation to step in and clear them away.

We also need to focus on and appreciate our good qualities. Without being able to recognize our good qualities, it would be difficult to cultivate them. In other words, we need to see the obscurations that we need to overcome, but we also need to cultivate the good qualities that we already have. It's very important to understand that our negative traits are not intrinsic: they *can* be eliminated, but they don't disappear by themselves. Just like some types of illnesses, negative traits develop due to temporary circumstances. At that point, the disease won't go away without some intervention. Using the analogy of disease, a doctor is necessary, some medicine is necessary, and some procedure is necessary. You can't skip any one of them. These interventions are factors conducive to healing. Likewise, we need teachers, explanations, and methods for eliminating obscurations and developing our compassion.

In order to be free of the "disease" of temporary obscurations, we first need the desire to be healthy—to be free of negative traits. Let's say that certain emotional states—greed, hatred, closed-minded-ness—are like seeds. We need to recognize what these seeds will grow into if allowed to flourish. If the fruits that these seeds eventually bore were beautiful, pleasant, and enjoyable, that would be fine. But they aren't. The fruits of negative emotions and actions are regarded as poisons—when you eat them, they make you sick. When you express those emotions, they make others unhappy. They immediately create a negative atmosphere and in the long run give rise to unhappiness and disaster. The will to be free of negative emotions comes from understanding that they produce these kinds of results. It's a very practical attitude.

The more that we are able to recognize and acknowledge the consequences of negative emotions, the more sincere our wish to develop loving kindness, compassion, and insight becomes. These positive emotions will come naturally, and we will also begin to develop more trust in their value and power. Trust means that we understand how they bring benefit, both immediately and in the long run. The more sincerely we appreciate the value of these qualities, the closer we are to manifesting those same noble qualities ourselves. If we truly want something, if we feel it is urgent, we put all our effort toward accomplishing that goal. We may forgo sleep, meals, anything, to realize our wish. The same holds true for our mind. The more we develop the will to be free of negative emotions, the more we appreciate noble qualities. This, in turn, makes our meditation training more sincere, and therefore more effective.

If we look as an outsider at the various activities of Tibetan Buddhist practitioners, we see people doing many different things. They might be putting flowers on a shrine or lighting candles at a sacred site. They might be joining their palms together in respect and bowing their heads to the ground in front of a teacher or a monument. They may be performing circumambulations of pilgrimage sites. Buddhists

engage in many different practices like this, not just silent meditation. If we investigate more closely, we can find out why are they doing
these things. Each gesture is symbolic and is a remedy to remove a
particular negative emotion. For example, making an offering is a
method to eliminate stinginess. Paying respect and bowing down is a
method to eliminate conceit and pride. Even something as apparently
straightforward as making an apology is a method to eliminate anger
and resentment. Each of the different practices has a particular purpose, and when used correctly, can be very effective.

Some of these gestures may look like the leftovers from a super-
stitious tradition. But these methods are effective antidotes for mental poisons. If performed with good motivation, there is no doubt they
work. Without investigating some of the more esoteric practices, we
can at least appreciate the value of apology. Apologizing is very beneficial in the spiritual sense, but also at a more mundane level. If you
have a misunderstanding or disharmony with a friend, if you apologize, it clears the air. It allows the bad feelings to evaporate. It may
be as simple as saying, "I'm sorry, I didn't really mean it." Misunder-
standings can develop even between quite close friends. You didn't
intentionally do something harmful, but inadvertently, or because you
got caught up in a negative emotion, you caused some trouble. Suddenly you are not getting along. Suddenly there is disharmony, hurt,
and suffering. What does it take to heal this situation? The best way
is to apologize.

There are many ways to apologize. If you just say "sorry" very
abruptly, without really meaning it, it will not work. Sometimes an
insincere apology is interpreted as even further criticism. What is the
best way to apologize? You need to speak from the bottom of your
heart. You need to express in your mind, in your words, and in your
actions the sincere wish for the other person to be happy. Even if the
action you are apologizing for is a serious breach, through sincere

apology you can completely heal the disharmony. You may even end up closer friends than before.

We all need to keep this in our heart, and apply it when needed. Emotions can be so powerful that even though we would like to apologize, it seems like we can't do it. It may take time. A day, a month, a year, sometimes a whole lifetime may go by without being able to apologize for something. It's very painful, very sad. Both sides suffer as a result. Apologizing is very powerful. It's also an example of using a good method to bring about a beneficial result.

The purpose of meditation is to eliminate negative traits in our mind and to promote our natural good qualities. This is the attitude that we should bring to our meditation practice. When we first begin meditating, it is practical to meditate with something held in mind. We may not be used to being completely open and spontaneous, holding nothing whatsoever in mind, completely free of a reference point. If we are not able to just be like that, it is more effective to practice while keeping an object of focus in mind.

The simplest thing to hold in mind is something neutral, like our breathing. Just noticing it, without thinking about it or analyzing it. When we focus on our breathing, we avoid drifting off into other thoughts and emotions. Just try to notice your breathing as the breath passes in and out of your nostrils. This doesn't require a lot of effort. Just naturally notice the movement of your breath. You don't need to analyze or control your breathing. Just notice how it feels—very relaxed, very natural. The main point is to remain mentally relaxed, in equanimity. You can stop reading for a few moments and try this.

What can we accomplish through this type of training? When we are meditating, we are not for or against anything, we're just noticing our breathing. Our attention is focused, but neutral. To the extent that we are able to string those moments together, we can achieve a sense of ease. A peaceful state of mind. That's the benefit.

As we sit and notice our breathing, we may notice that our thoughts have strayed. It may be a memory of something that happened in the past, or perhaps something that we're planning for the future. We may have been distracted by something taking place at the present moment. In each case, we've been thinking about something other than our breathing. When we notice that we're distracted, we need to remind ourselves to go back to just noticing our breathing, again and again. We don't need to be hard on ourselves—after all we are practicing to learn how to be completely relaxed. We just need to redirect the mind back to the breath over and over, as many times as necessary. Since the mind is normally very active and easily distracted, this may not come so easily, but it becomes easier and easier. Practice makes perfect. The more we train, the simpler it gets.

At a certain point we may be able to keep our attention focused on the sensation of breathing for fifteen minutes without it wandering off. If we get really, really good at this, it's possible to remain for a whole hour completely at peace. There is a saying from the Buddha: unless your attention remains calm, you don't see clearly. This seeing clearly is actually a very profound point. That's the essence of wisdom, the clear insight that is free of concepts. There is a way of knowing in which we conceptualize, and there is a way of knowing in which there is no forming of concepts.

This thought-free wakefulness that sees clearly is the quintessence of Buddhist spiritual practice. First we need to recognize exactly how that is, then we train in it until it becomes totally stable. Stability in thought-free wakefulness is the same as complete liberation. The complete cessation of all negative traits allows our positive qualities to manifest naturally. Effortless compassion is one of the qualities that manifests from thought-free wakefulness.

Thought-free wakefulness is both empty and awake at the same time. *Empty* means there is nothing to pinpoint, like open space. At the same time there is an awake quality of being present to whatever is. These two qualities, being empty and awake, sound as if they are two separate things that have been united, but it's not like that at all. They are indivisible. Just like the example of water and its quality of being wet—they cannot be separated. This unity of being empty and awake is unformed, unconstructed. Everything formed will perish, but this basic nature is unformed.

Meditation Instruction

I will now give some more formal instructions on how to practice the type of meditation that utilizes the breath as a focus. Simply agreeing that we need to meditate does not produce any real effect. The theory may be very clear in our minds, and we may be able to enumerate a host of benefits, but as long as it is just a theory, it will not help us. The only way to progress in relaxation is by training. We should try it for ourselves and see if there is a benefit.

We begin by arranging our body. When it comes to posture, the most important point is to keep your back straight. It shouldn't be tense or rigid, but it should be stable and straight, with the shoulders relaxed. If you can sit with crossed legs, that's fine. If you are already in the habit of sitting cross-legged, then this will not be difficult. There are reasons that Buddhists prefer to sit in the cross-legged position, but if that is difficult for you, it is perfectly fine to sit in a chair. The way we sit is just a matter of habit, isn't it? When I flew to America on an airplane, at first I sat with my legs down on the floor. As time went on, that position became uncomfortable for me, so I ended up sitting cross-legged on the airplane seat. The person next to me gave me a funny look—he thought I was a little strange. But it's just a matter of habit.

So you need a straight back, but relaxed. You can put your hands together comfortably in your lap, palms up, with your left hand on the bottom, and the fingers of your right hand resting just on top of the fingers of your left hand. The tips of your thumbs then gently touch each other, forming a circle. This is called the gesture of peace. It's also fine to just rest your hands on your thighs. If your aim initially is to train in being calm, then it's better to close the eyes, because if you have your eyes open, you will start to think about all the things in your line of vision. But ultimately the real practice is not merely to feel calm, but to be at peace in a way that is open and vast.

Once you have positioned the body so that it is stable and relaxed, direct your attention toward the movement of the breath. Feel the breath moving through the nostrils. Try to keep your attention fixed on the movement of your breath, sensing the motion at the opening of the nostrils. The mind will naturally wander, for that is its present habit. But with practice, continually bringing the attention back to the breath over and over, you will come to notice more quickly that the mind has wandered, and your concentration will grow stronger.

Over the course of a training session, your nature changes slightly. You have the experience of being more calm, more quiet. As you finish your training session and stand up and move about, it seems that your mental state has changed a bit. You feel less disturbed and more steady. That is the effect of this training. I think we can all agree that this is something worthwhile.

When you sit down to do this meditation, there's no need to recall what happened in the past, no need to make plans for the future. In each passing moment, there's no need to form thoughts about what you feel, see, hear, or about any other sense impressions. There's only one thing you need to be concerned with, and that is the neutral sensation of the breath passing through your nostrils. Just notice it as it happens. You don't need to do anything at all other than that. Just relax in a state of equanimity, simply noticing the breathing. It's important not to do anything contrived. You are already breathing—just notice it. When you exhale, exhale normally, not trying to exhale; when inhaling, just inhale like you normally do. You don't have to consciously control your breathing. Simply notice.

You may find that your attention does not remain full-time on your breathing. One moment you are watching your breath, and then you notice that your attention has drifted off. Even without wanting to start thinking of something else, it happens. Isn't that true? What you are training in during breath meditation is noticing when the attention drifts off from the breath and bringing your attention back to the breath, over and over again. That's the training. We can call it *meditation,* but I personally prefer the word *training*. We can think of it as training in being calm.

When we first start training in being calm, it is more practical to direct the attention at something like our breath in order to avoid thinking of other things. However, as I've already mentioned, that is not our ultimate goal. After spending time growing more settled by focusing on our inhalation and exhalation in a very simple, neutral way, we discover that it is possible to be calm and present without concentrating on an object. At that point, rather than focusing on something, we are simply calm and present, very open, without deliberately holding anything in mind. Just very open, very present, but also settled. After training like that for a while, at some point we discover a state of complete openness, wherein awareness does not fixate or make concepts about anything whatsoever. It's a very alive, vivid state that is empty like space yet very awake—free of forming concepts but not blind or dull in any way. That is what is meant by *thought-free wakefulness*. It is our basic nature, simply as it is.

When we first gain this experience of our basic nature, that's called *recognizing*. Just having had a glimpse of this recognition is not enough after a while. We need to train in it by experiencing it over and over again. That's how its strength grows and becomes perfected.

Ultimately, even that is not enough. We finally reach a point at which we no longer waver from that state of awake openness. In other words, we gain complete stability. That's our ultimate goal.

As our training progresses, we notice that our tendencies to be blindly attached, angry, closed-minded, and so forth, begin to diminish. They don't hold so much power any longer. The noble qualities that I have explained—being compassionate, caring, and so forth—arise more spontaneously. Finally, when the negative traits have vanished completely and the noble qualities arise unceasingly, there is total stability in the state of uncontrived naturalness. It is now completely effortless. That is called being enlightened, being a buddha. It's not something other than that.

12

Learning to Monitor
Our Mental State

THE KEY TO EXPERIENCING COMPASSION that arises naturally is creating a relaxed state of mind. However, there are also other techniques that help to expand compassion toward others. These techniques involve adopting progressive stages of a compassionate attitude. The first stage is to try to stop thinking of ourselves as being more important than others. The second stage is to try to mentally put ourselves in another's place—to be willing to exchange ourselves with others. The third stage is to regard others as more important than ourselves.

We cannot start off regarding others as more important than ourselves because it is very difficult to do. That's why we begin with the first two stages. The third stage of compassion has as its basis a profound sense of love and affection. Most mothers experience the third stage of compassion when they have a child, when, for the most part, a mother regards her baby as more important than herself. Most mothers don't experience this attitude before having a baby. Until the baby comes along, a woman may feel that her own feelings and safety are paramount. However, as soon as the baby is born, there is a spontaneous shift in the mother's attitude, wherein the baby becomes the more important person. A mother's (or father's) feeling for a child is a

very good example of the attitude we are striving for in the third stage
in cultivating compassion.

What causes this change in the mother's or father's attitude? There
must be a reason. The reason is love and affection. A very strong feeling of love and caring on the part of the parents arises in response to
their child, something very pure. What makes it pure? It is the fact
that the mother or father is not expecting anything back from the
baby. That's a very important point. For when love expects a reward,
it may appear to be pure love, but actually it's more like a business
transaction.

People are always talking about love—love between friends, love
between couples. People who care about each other often say, "I love
you." They say this when they feel very close to one another. But what
does love really mean? We need to investigate a little more deeply. We
may not know what pure love really is. When two people think they
are very much in love they often say to each other, "I love you very
much." However, sooner or later, one person may discover that what
they are really in love with is not the other person, but the pleasurable feeling they get from their attraction to the other person. When the
feeling of attraction diminishes, the feeling of love subsides as well. If
the attraction disappears, the love disappears. That's very sad.

What this means is that the love was not pure. Sometimes couples
who think they really love each other discover a problem in their relationship. They slowly begin to experience difficulties. They start to
bicker. If they can't resolve the problem, they may try to get help from
a therapist. Maybe the ostensible problem is a small thing: one person
wants to go hiking, and the other person says, "I hate hiking." The
issue is small, but it is a symptom that perhaps they are not getting
along well. What is the basis of the relationship? Is it love? Or is it
need? If the relationship is rooted in need, then whenever the need for
the other person is reduced, love is reduced.

Love needs to be based on care and respect. If love is based on genuine care and respect, then that type of love is very pure, very stable. You could call it "unshakable love." If love is based on attraction or need, however, that love is fragile and shallow. A mother's love for a child is an example of unshakable love. The mother is not wishing or hoping for a reward from the child. She's not saying, "I wish just once my child would make me a cup of coffee!"

Through this powerful feeling of love, the mother automatically learns patience. Through love she learns diligence. Through love she learns concentration. Through love she learns what it means to be aware. Wherever the child is, the mother will know. The mother may be having a conversation with you, but part of her thoughts are on the child. Part of her mind is always tracking the movements of the child. All of this awareness, patience, diligence, and concentration comes from a pure feeling of love toward the child. Whatever important business the mother needs to carry on, whatever the occasion, the mother will not forget for even one second that she is responsible for her child. In the Tibetan language we call that quality *drenpa,* which means mindfulness.

Spiritual practitioners need to develop mindfulness of their own mental state that is as powerful as a mother's mindfulness of her child's well-being. You could say that the mother's mindfulness of her child's welfare is rarely interrupted. If the child is a small baby, the mother is constantly thinking about it. What is the baby doing? Is it hungry? Is it thirsty? Is it cold? Is it fine? And so forth. She gives the child unceasing attention. It is that degree of attention, of paying attention, that a spiritual practitioner needs.

In order to eventually be able to influence our mental state for the better, we first need to be able to monitor what is taking place in our own mind. Are the thoughts negative or positive? What is our attitude at any given moment? However, just monitoring our mental state will not bring about change. We need to be able to switch directions if we are in a negative frame of mind. That is possible. We *can* switch directions—we can change a negative mental state into something neutral, or even-minded. We can then change that even-minded state into something wholesome and noble. That is possible. But having a noble attitude is still not sufficient, because even with a noble attitude there's still some sense of clinging, though it may be very subtle. Whenever our attention clings to something—holds a concept in mind—we create a platform upon which negative emotions can return and start to accumulate.

The primary cause of negative emotions, no matter what kind they are, is a deviation of our attention away from our natural state of empty awareness toward a state in which we form thoughts and emotions about what we are seeing. This is what is described as dualistic thinking. Understanding dualistic thinking is necessary in order to know the root cause of all our suffering. Therefore, rather than just dismissing this as being beyond our understanding, it is useful to think, "Could this be true? Is there a way for me to understand this?"

You should continue to investigate duality until you have no doubt whether it is true or not. If you just read these words and vaguely agree that this could be a plausible theory of consciousness, it's not the same as becoming certain about it for yourselves. Each individual needs to personally resolve this issue if they are to develop a true understanding, and the best way to eliminate doubt is through investigation.

Once you develop a firm conviction based on thorough investigation, you can then use mindfulness to monitor how well you are integrating that insight into the rest of your life. If that mindfulness has been developed so that it is as strong as a mother's vigilance for the welfare of her baby, then you will make swift progress in overcoming negative emotions and expanding your wisdom and compassion so that they are without limit.

13

The Qualities of
an Authentic Teacher

I N THE BUDDHIST TRADITION, great importance is placed on finding
the right teacher to help guide you to your goals. I have mentioned
earlier that even though our basic nature is inherent in all of us, we are
unable to recognize our basic nature without the help of a teacher.
The wrong teacher could lead us in unsuitable directions, so it is
important to reflect on what makes an authentic teacher. *Authenticity*
refers to something that we can verify as real, a description of how
things actually are. In the Buddhist context, it refers to someone who
is free of all flaws or faults, and endowed with all perfect qualities.
That is the definition of truly authentic. A truly authentic teacher is
called a *buddha*. There have been many buddhas in the past, there are
buddhas in the present, and there will be more in the future. The
"present Buddha" refers to the buddha of our times, Buddha Shakyamuni, who began his life as Prince Siddhartha and taught the Dharma
in India over 2,500 years ago.

When we say that a buddha is free of flaws, what kind of flaws are
we talking about? The flaws are the two obscurations and the habitual tendencies, which I introduced briefly in chapter 7. An obscuration is anything that covers our basic nature. The first obscuration is
the *emotional obscuration,* meaning getting angry, attached, proud,

jealous, closed-minded, and so forth. Buddhism says there are 84,000 different variations of these negative emotions. To be totally free of *all* of these negative emotions is to be free of the emotional obscuration. The second obscuration is called *cognitive obscuration,* which is the forming of concepts about what we experience. These concepts form a barrier between what we perceive and the actual nature of things. The cognitive obscuration prevents true wisdom. *Habitual tendencies* refers to the fact that even though we may be free of these two obscurations for a brief period through spiritual practice, the tendency for them to come back is still there. The pattern lingers on, just as our dreams at night tend to carry on with what we have experienced emotionally during the day.

A truly authentic teacher—a buddha—is not just free of faults. To be truly authentic, certain qualities must be present. These qualities are called the *twofold sublime knowledge.* The first knowledge is the ability to see the true nature of things exactly as they are. The other knowledge is the ability, while remaining in the recognition of one's unconditioned basic nature, to know whatever possibly exists at any time and in any place.

What is encompassed by "whatever possibly exists"? It doesn't mean just one world or one universe. The domain over which a buddha is able to sustain awareness encompasses one billion simultaneous universes. The universes are not all at the same stage of evolution. Some are in the process of expanding, some have fully expanded and will remain for some time, some are in the process of contracting, and some have contracted and completely vanished. One billion universes, all at different stages.

In each universe there are countless sentient beings, all of them different—different shapes, different characters, different inclinations, different stages of birth and death. They engage in different karmic actions that become the causes of the various life forms, their states of mind, and their emotions. The exact situation of each of those sentient beings in all of those universes is known without obstruction in the awakened state of a buddha, each arising completely unmixed and distinct from all others.

Along with being able to see the delusions of each sentient being, a buddha is also able to perceive the potential for being a buddha that is inherent in each being. Even though sentient beings are temporarily beset by the two obscurations, they still have the innate ability to be totally pure, because their basic nature is identical to that of a buddha. A buddha also knows how to help guide each of those sentient beings toward recognizing their own true nature. All of these qualities added together is called "knowing what possibly exists." Taken together, these two qualities—knowing the true nature of things, and knowing all that possibly exists—can be called *omniscience*.

As you can see, incredible qualities are present in the awakened state of a buddha. There are additional qualities as well. The physical presence of a buddha is completely pleasing to anyone. One never tires of looking at him or her. The body is free of any flaws; the voice is perfect in various ways. When speaking, the voice does not halt or pause to figure out what to say next. Each syllable is distinct and has meaning and carries pleasing qualities to the listener. When listening to a buddha teach, it makes no difference whether you sit close or far away, you can still hear very clearly. There are no extraneous sounds mixed in like "uh," or "mmm." The teachings are spoken with perfect intonation. Each person can understand what is being said in his or her own language, without the need for a translator.

We need to remember that the perfect qualities that we are discussing are not limited to this one person who lived long ago in India. Whoever has purified their individual flaws—the two obscurations and habitual tendencies—and whoever has allowed their qualities of compassion to be fully manifest, is a perfect teacher, male or female.

To put it simply, whoever has awakened from ignorance and perfected wisdom is an awakened one, a buddha.

I am aware that this must sound pretty unbelievable. It's not really possible to grasp with the rational mind. Words are not adequate to describe some situations. Just as it is impossible to measure the size of outer space by using a tape measure, our normal intellect can fail to understand some vast concepts. Recognizing all the qualities that are associated with our basic nature—which we call *buddha nature*—defies the efforts of rational thought. However, just because we can't measure all of space with a tape measure doesn't mean that space is limited to the small part that we *can* measure.

A buddha is not just awakened or realized, but is motivated and capable of teaching a path for sentient beings to become enlightened themselves. Right now we do not have the opportunity to meet the historical Buddha, the buddha of our era. But of all the enlightened qualities of the Buddha, there is still one that can affect us right now, and that is the words that were spoken. The words of the Buddha exist in about one hundred huge volumes. In addition to those basic texts, the great masters of the centuries that followed after the Buddha wrote further explanations and treatises, of which there are thousands.

The words of the Buddha and the commentaries of the great masters are still available. The Buddha also gave instructions on how to utilize these teachings. The Buddha felt that the teachings themselves were well spoken and perfect. However, he made it clear that no one is required to believe these teachings without first checking them for themselves. The words of a buddha that are available are something beneficial, perfect, and very pure. Although someone like myself may already be convinced, each of us is encouraged to question the value of what is being taught, to test it for ourselves, before we decide whether it is valid or not. Not only is it acceptable to examine the validity and worth of the teachings for ourselves, we are actively *encouraged* to do so. After that we are free to choose to accept the teachings or not.

The qualities of the awakened mind of a buddha are innumerable. But all of these qualities can be summed up in two words: wisdom and compassion. Wisdom has the qualities of knowledge that I've already discussed. What is enlightened compassion like? It is impartial, makes no distinction between friend or enemy, close or distant. There is no bias, no prejudice whatsoever. In other words, if someone makes offerings to a buddha and bows down, it makes no difference to the buddha. If another person hurls abuse or tries to strike a buddha, it also makes no difference. The sense of caring for the other person's welfare doesn't waver. This kind of compassion can be called *nonconceptual compassion,* expressing itself as impartial love or effortless love.

Nonconceptual compassion means we are able to act without first having made the decision to do so. Nonconceptual compassion is the natural expression of having realized our basic nature. It's a way of caring or affection that is spontaneous, natural, and effortless. It does not rely on our having decided whether to be compassionate in a given situation.

Buddhas are not necessarily far away in space or time. There is no law that prohibits any sentient being from being a buddha. Why? Because, as I have said, we all have exactly the same nature that can be uncovered, and the same qualities that can be revealed. The seed for being a buddha is present in everyone. Not just human beings— animals, insects, and whatever life forms there are—all have buddha nature within. The nature of that fundamental consciousness is identical with that of a fully enlightened buddha.

What determines whether a sentient being becomes a buddha or not? Progress on the path to full enlightenment depends on both the right circumstances and the right effort. Right now our basic nature, what is sometimes called the *unconditioned suchness,* is present within us like a seed. Like a seed, it requires the right circumstances to grow. When the right circumstances are present, the seed can begin to grow. When the right circumstances are continually present, the seed can grow into a fully bloomed flower.

Similarly, the right circumstances are necessary to allow our buddha nature to fully manifest. In the example of the flower, the circumstances need to be conducive to growth. Simply having pretty or expensive surroundings is not conducive. If you put a flower seed into a box made of gold and decorated with silver and diamonds, for example, it won't help it grow. For a seed you need soil, water, and fertilizer, the right temperature, enough room to grow, sufficient time, and so forth. Whenever these circumstances come together in the right combination, the seed does not hesitate. It grows instant by instant. We know that a fully developed flower looks beautiful, and may smell very nice. But it takes time, and the right circumstances, for a flower to develop fully and be able to provide enjoyment for whoever sees it.

The meaning of this example is that everyone—all sentient beings—have the potential, the seed, the nature of being a buddha. This potential is always present, all of the time. In every sesame seed there is always oil potentially present. In milk there is always butter potentially present. But if you don't press the sesame seed, you don't get the oil. If you don't churn the milk and apply some effort, you don't get any butter. In the same way, unless we supply the conducive circumstances, and get rid of whatever it is that prevents us from directly experiencing our true nature, it just doesn't become evident or visible. Therefore, we need some education and training. We need to first study the words of an awakened being, someone who has already realized their basic nature. Next we need to reflect on the meaning of the teachings until we really understand them. Once we really understand, then we need to apply the teachings in our lives.

This process is known as developing the understanding that comes from learning, reflection, and meditation. Learning and reflection allow us to get the theory. Getting the theory is important, but it is not enough. No matter how clearly we get the theory, it's not sufficient to remove the obscurations and the habitual tendencies and to allow the qualities of knowledge to really blossom. We need something more, and that is the knowledge that comes through actual experience. That is why training in meditation is so important. The end result is that we greatly reduce our negative tendencies and vastly increase our positive qualities—like a buddha.

14

Examples of Enlightened Resolve

ANYONE WHO IS TRAINING to be more compassionate needs to have examples to emulate. That is true within the Buddhist tradition as well. I'd like to introduce you to a brave type of person who pledges to take care of not just a few, but all sentient beings. This pledge includes not just the people he or she actually meets, but is a resolve to care for all sentient beings equally. In other words, such a person has vowed to move toward awakening out of compassion for others. Forming that resolve takes a lot of courage. Such a person is called a *bodhisattva*, and the resolve is called *bodhichitta*, which means "enlightened resolve."

A bodhisattva sets out to conquer selfish emotions and to perfect his or her enlightened qualities. A bodhisattva is fearless, unafraid of how many beings there may be, how many eons it may take, or how difficult it may be. That's a pretty good definition of brave, isn't it? Once the resolve is clearly formed, such a person can begin to take action out of that resolve. That is called the bodhisattva activity.

A bodhisattva has all-encompassing compassion and kindness. Although this may sound difficult to achieve, it is possible for any individual to increase the two noble qualities of loving-kindness and compassion. It requires effort on our part, but it is possible. We can become better at being loving and compassionate by gradually expanding the range of beings included, wider and wider, until no one is excluded. The goal is to ultimately have compassion that is completely impartial or unbiased. Accomplishing that goal is a real possibility. We can make up our mind to awaken our own bodhichitta, to train in developing the pure attitude of a bodhisattva.

Training to be a bodhisattva is based on developing six major virtues. The first virtue is generosity. What does generosity mean in the context of practicing medicine? It means the willingness to give whatever is necessary—not just the medicine or the treatment, but to be there in a way that comforts the sick person. In your behavior, in your speech, and in your heart, you feel directly or indirectly willing to do whatever is necessary. It is a generous way of being that is not superficial, but is genuine and sincere. That is the meaning of generosity here.

The second virtue is pure ethics. What does that mean in relation to the practice of medicine? It means developing a highly conscientious attitude that allows you to be concerned about your patients in the right way. Pure ethics means developing the instincts to do the right thing on the spot, whatever it is that needs to be done. It means you don't put off doing the right thing because you are tired or lazy. If you cultivate a genuine feeling of caring for others, the sense of wanting to help can be increased right away. That is the meaning of ethics in this context: to be conscientious and to try to avoid being careless or feeling frustrated.

The third virtue of a bodhisattva is tolerance. Tolerance is necessary because patients sometimes become exasperated. They may feel that they are just not getting cured fast enough, especially if their illness or treatment is particularly unpleasant or painful. They may have placed all their hope in the doctor, and start to feel that the doctor is just not making them better fast enough. They begin to think they can't take it any longer, and may begin to resent the doctor. Some patients may not only start to feel that way, they may actually become physically violent. They may suddenly try to hit the doctor or nurse, or lash out with verbal abuse. They may say truly awful things, not because it makes sense to do so, but because they have become irrational. A patient may become so aggressive, annoying, and irritating that you start to think, "What am I doing here? I've tried my best, but there's no gratitude from this person. I give up. Let someone else deal with this."

That is the point at which your tolerance has finally slipped. You don't have to let it go that far. You can understand that it is not personal at all. The patient is acting from a state of desperation that has very little to do with the particular doctor or nurse. The patient has a distorted point of view—the despair that they feel displays itself as aggression. It's very important to understand this, because otherwise you simply want to send that patient somewhere else—to another doctor, to another section of the hospital, or even to another hospital. Whatever it takes to get the patient out from under your care. You think, "I don't want to deal with that person anymore. He's impossible." This way of thinking not only demonstrates a lack of tolerance, it's unwise. Such an attitude simply reflects that you have not been able to see things from the patient's perspective.

I'm not suggesting that you shouldn't refer the patient when it is appropriate. If you truly believe that another opinion or more specialized care will benefit the patient, then that referral comes from positive motivation. But if you are acting out of fatigue, frustration, or anger, and simply don't want to care for that particular person any more, that is not good motivation. If the motivation is not good, the tolerance will soon be gone, the compassion will be gone, and eventually the patient will be gone.

The fourth virtue is perseverance. Perseverance is the willingness to carry through to the end of the treatment. That can be done in various ways. We can persevere unwillingly, not because we *want* to help, but because we feel we have no choice—it's our job. You carry on with a vague feeling of "I have to do it, so I'll do it." Alternatively, perseverance could be accomplished with a sense of joy. You could think, "I want to see that person cured," and then carry through with that attitude. The term for this kind of perseverance is *joyous diligence.*

Joyous diligence comes from pure motivation, a kind of perfect willingness to help. To help develop that kind of motivation, you can reflect in this way on the suffering that the patient is going through: "Whoever is suffering has pain. If I suffer, I have pain. If somebody took care of me and helped me, I'd be very grateful and happy. Now this person has come to me with high expectations, so I will do my best to help. I will take whatever action is needed with my body, speech, and mind. I'll use whatever medicine or equipment is necessary. I'll look in my books if I need to. I'll use all my skill, purely and diligently." This type of diligence is based on taking joy in your efforts.

It's important to realize that whatever you take joy in doesn't tend to make you feel tired. You can carry on much longer with an activity that is satisfying and gives you joy. Honestly, the job of healing is something intrinsically good. It helps relieve suffering. Someone has a problem, and you are able to offer your services. It's wonderful. Therefore, it's reasonable to imagine that you could take pleasure in the activity of healing.

The fifth and the sixth virtues are usually discussed in the context of meditation practice, but that doesn't mean we can't also apply the principles to the art of healing. The fifth virtue is cultivating pure concentration. That means paying attention, not allowing yourself to get distracted from what you are doing. This is very applicable to the medical profession. If you are supposed to be dealing with a serious problem, it's not a good idea to start thinking of something totally unrelated. If you are able to concentrate, then you can avoid careless errors. To practice medicine properly, one needs to pay attention, to be mindful, and to be focused on the present situation. An example of not paying attention in a concentrated way is when you write a note that the right leg is injured when you mean the left leg. Or you describe the condition of one patient in the chart of another by mistake. There are many possible examples. The intent is not evil. The error is the result of being distracted when you should be paying attention. That's why we need the fifth virtue, concentration.

The sixth virtue is actually the most important of all. The sixth virtue is to be intelligent in a very specific sense. Maintaining that specific sense of intelligence is necessary while practicing all of the virtues. You need an intelligent generosity, intelligent ethics, intelligent tolerance, intelligent perseverance, and intelligent concentration. Intelligence in this context refers to an awake quality—the ability to see the situation clearly. This intelligence—or wisdom—is based on viewing things in an open-minded way, not obscured by preconceived ideas.

One major obstacle that can prevent seeing clearly might be intellectual or professional pride. Educated people who have positions of responsibility, such as professors, doctors, or politicians, are supposed to be competent. Some of them will listen to an array of suggestions before making a decision—they are comfortable consulting with other people. Others in positions of responsibility, however, may have the attitude of not wanting to listen to others, confident that their own opinion is best. Once they have made up their mind, they don't want to consult anyone else. This attitude could come from pride, or it could stem from a sense of rivalry with others. There are numerous reasons for feeling like that. But we don't have to give in to that tendency. If this attitude is present, it may be wisest to not simply follow that pattern, but instead be more open-minded. We need to be willing to find what is best, rather than just assuming we already know.

Doctors generally start out with similar training. However, over time your own experiences and insights may become quite different from

another doctor. Therefore, it makes sense to discuss problems with
other professionals. You could find that light is suddenly shed on a
previously difficult situation. When professionals are willing to discuss a problem with their peers, it can be truly beneficial.

To summarize, *bodhichitta* means the enlightened or awakened
frame of mind, which is motivated by the sincere wish to help others.
The relationship between bodhichitta and the natural state is that
when we are resting in our natural state, there is a spontaneous benevolence, without any concepts. Bodhichitta is naturally and completely
present, without any contrived aspects. The direct experience of the
natural state is called the *absolute* or *ultimate bodhichitta*. Conversely,
whenever we consciously feel that we want to help others, that is
called the *relative bodhichitta*. By cultivating and training in relative
bodhichitta, we can eventually realize the ultimate awakened state.
That's the connection. As long as we haven't recognized the natural
state, then the kindness and compassion we have is considered relative. Once we have recognized the natural state, then there is spontaneous kindness, and we experience absolute bodhichitta. All we
need to start this process is enlightened resolve.

15

The Need for a Teacher

Buddhist teachings always emphasize that a teacher is necessary to help us recognize our basic nature. Some people may feel that they can discover this basic essence by themselves. However, we should be able to agree that training in something very important usually requires a teacher. Are people able to become doctors without teachers? Is it possible that say 99 percent of medical students have had teachers, and 1 percent have had none? It just doesn't happen that way. If you try to treat patients without studying medicine with a qualified doctor, you cannot be effective at helping them. If that weren't true, it would be easy to help others. Whenever we encountered sick people we could just automatically know how to make them better.

Isn't it also true that to be allowed to teach medical students, you have to be competent? Not just anybody can walk in and be the educator of doctors. The medical school professor must have specific qualifications. Thus, you need not only a teacher to learn how to practice medicine properly, you need a qualified teacher. And to be able to help students in the best possible way, a teacher needs to set a good example. If a medical professor is not only knowledgeable about medicine, but also patient, tolerant, and generous, the students will respond well. If, however, the teacher knows a lot about medical topics but does not have much patience and acts irritable and abrupt, it makes the students uneasy.

Beyond a teacher, you also need patients—people who are suffering and require some care. One cannot get by with just knowing the theory. Personal experience in treating patients is required. If you had no patients, how would you gain experience? Similarly, while proceeding along the spiritual path, you train in being generous, ethical, tolerant, and so forth. And in order to be able to cultivate these qualities, you need other beings to interact with. Just as you need both a good teacher and patients to cultivate the qualities of a good doctor, in Buddhist training you need both buddhas and sentient beings, and by means of both you can make spiritual progress.

In the Buddhist context, the word "teacher" is not synonymous with "spiritual guide." To be a teacher, you can just study the theory, and when you are able to repeat it skillfully, they call you a teacher. However, that is not enough to be considered a spiritual guide. In order to guide someone else, you must have knowledge based on personal experience. You need a taste of genuine experience, because the spiritual guide is not someone who just imparts theory. It's his or her responsibility to guide someone else toward experiences that they have personally realized, not just toward a theoretical ideal. Therefore, the spiritual guide must have some realization and compassion. When these two qualities are present, the person can be called a qualified spiritual guide.

However, just having a qualified teacher or guide is not sufficient. The person on the receiving end also needs to be qualified. The medical professor may be a great teacher, but if the students are uninterested or incapable of learning, they won't become good doctors. To learn to be a doctor, the most important quality is a genuine desire to be a doctor. To attain spiritual progress, you need a similar kind of desire. You could call it sincerity, interest, or trust. You also need perseverance that will carry you through not just the study of theory, but through the acquisition of practical experience as well. I mentioned earlier that proper perseverance is not just forcing one-self through the training, but understanding the value of what one is undertaking, and therefore embracing it with a sense of joy. This joyous diligence is especially important when you are trying to gain practical experience.

In spiritual training, as in medical training, if you stop halfway, with just intellectual understanding, there's some risk. In spiritual train-ing, unless you bring the theory into practice, it won't have a genuine effect on you, and it won't eradicate your personal shortcomings. If you don't use the instructions to truly integrate theory and practice, it is easy to become conceited, or proud, because you have achieved some theoretical understanding. When you are all puffed up because of some intellectual learning, you tend to automatically regard others as being less important than yourself. You may be tempted to belittle someone else's understanding. Actually undergoing spiritual training, or attempting to care for real patients, is inherently humbling.

However, once you begin to integrate your intellectual under-standing with personal experience, something begins to happen. A certain appreciation and trust and compassion begin to arise sponta-neously. You develop a deeper appreciation of the instructions and the spiritual or medical guide. Why does that happen? Because you start to feel that you are changing—that some real insight and confidence is developing. You realize that this change has come directly from applying a particular instruction. In that way you begin to appreciate the value of the instruction and the person who is the source of the instruction. You begin to trust in your training because the teachings and practice have had an actual effect on yourself, or on the care of your patients. By appreciating how *we* have been able to change, we become more aware of the capacity for change that must also exist in others. This allows compassion for others to gradually increase.

By studying the theory behind Buddhist practice, you become more aware of the qualities that can be developed through spiritual practice. Based on these descriptions, you begin to admire those who have perfected these practices, and you develop a longing to be like that yourself. That's why we study the theory. When the theory becomes actual experience, the good qualities begin to unfold in you. Blind and deluded traits diminish, and your confidence in spiritual practice increases. At a certain point that confidence can become unshakable. When you just study the theory, this type of unshakable confidence can't develop. You gain merely an idea of how things could be. When you actually experience it yourself, that's a different feeling.

Before we are able to gain some experience in seeing the natural state of mind, we can, of course, feel compassion. We might even feel spontaneous compassion for friends and loved ones. But it still requires effort to feel compassion for strangers. We have to try harder to be nice to people that we don't know. When it comes to people who have hurt us, then it becomes really difficult. Even if we try to act with compassion in those circumstances, we don't really feel it. The best we can do is to fake it a little bit.

When we begin to assimilate the real spiritual practice of knowing our basic nature, the barriers to compassion are no longer so rigid. Compassion becomes more open, more free, requiring less effort. It's easier to feel close or affectionate toward anyone we meet because we don't have the same conceptual barriers. Even when you meet someone who has apparently tried to hurt you or your feelings, it won't disturb you that much, and you can still be kind to them. These are some of the qualities generated by the insight we gain from practical training, based on the instructions from a teacher.

16

Different Kinds of Teachers

A s I mentioned in the last chapter, a teacher is necessary in order to make progress along the spiritual path. We may not be able to personally meet and take teachings from an authentic teacher when we first become interested in spiritual development. However, in the Buddhist tradition there are four kinds of teachers. By knowing how to take advantage of these resources, we can start on the spiritual path without delay.

The first kind of teacher consists of the words of enlightened beings. This is valuable advice in written form, transcribed from the teachings of enlightened masters of the past, such as the historical Buddha and others. When we study and assimilate the meaning from written words, we get some guidance. In this sense, the written word is a way of receiving teachings. But the author has to be someone who is both wise and kind. The best authors, of course, are those that are said to be free from ignorance. In Buddhist thought, it is said that he or she has awakened from their blind spots.

In a story from the time of the Buddha, a teenager came to the Buddha and said, "Who are you actually? A lot of people talk about you, and your name is heard here and there, but who are you really?" The Buddha replied, "I am the awakened one." If an awakened being is the author, then what is written down directly from that person's teachings is authentic and correct. That's one type of teacher.

The second type of teacher is called a living lineage teacher, the holder of knowledge that has been passed on through an unbroken lineage of people. A master instructs a student with oral instructions on what to avoid and what to adopt in order to gain insight. That student, once having fully realized the teachings for him or herself, passes them on to the next person. In fact, these oral instructions have been passed on from one person to the next, from the original teachings of the Buddha until the present time. The one who is last in this line is someone whom we can actually meet and take advice from. We call that kind of teacher a living lineage teacher.

Such a person, of course, needs to have many qualifications. He or she needs to be well versed in philosophy and other written teachings, but also needs to be accomplished in the experiential sense. From the Buddhist point of view, this person—who can be male or female—needs to have personal experience in what I previously described as "compassionate emptiness." That is the baseline. *Emptiness* in this context can also be called "intelligent insight." No one can teach someone else how to achieve this state of mind without first stabilizing it within themselves. When a teacher has the intelligent insight into the state of emptiness, that person is free of ignorance, is free of unknowing.

Insight into emptiness also dissolves the ignorant clinging to duality, which allows true compassion to manifest. The atmosphere of openness that occurs when we do not cling to any concepts allows for unlimited, nonconceptual compassion to become evident. A clean and pure compassion unfolds within that atmosphere of openness—a form of compassion that is not prejudiced or limited in any way. As soon as the ignorant clinging to duality dissolves, the compassion that results is like a mother's care for her only child, applied to anyone you meet. A person who manifests this type of compassionate emptiness can truly be called a living lineage master.

A third type of teacher is the symbolic teacher of experiences, which consists of the experiences that we have in our daily lives. We all have a wide variety of experiences that lead us to feel many different emotions. However, these experiences all pass behind us and vanish as they occur. The whole thing that we think of as "my life" is, in actuality, something very ethereal and hard to describe.

The Buddha said that the world is impermanent and fleeting like autumn clouds. In India, where he lived, the cloud formations in the autumn sky change very fast. Similarly, the birth and death of beings is said to be like watching a drama on a stage. In a play, whole lifetimes might be played out within an hour or two—someone is born, grows up, and dies. The birth and death of beings is like watching a dramatic performance. Our happy and sad times can be our teachers, we can learn from them, learn from the drama we are enacting. Even facing illness and death can be seen as a learning experience.

Doctors usually relate to disease as something that affects the patient, not themselves. But doctors are basically no different than patients. Doctors can fall ill as well. Due to the nature of their work, doctors may witness a lot of death. If they are honest with themselves, they will admit that they are standing in that same line—waiting in line to die. That's difficult to contemplate. What can you do when confronted with a death? You can utilize these events as teachers. What we need to learn from these experiences is how to be good at living while we are alive. If we fall ill, we need to know how to be good at being ill—how to make the best of it. When we begin to die, we also need to be good at dying.

It's especially important to be an expert at dying. If people didn't die, then there would be no use in talking about that subject. Why bother talking about dying if there is a chance that we won't die? However, if we look around we can't find any examples of people who have not died. If we were able to meet in this world just one person who has not died, or is not destined to die, or if we just heard that such a person might exist, then we could begin to have doubt about whether we ourselves would have to die. Even if there were just one person like that, then we could think, "Maybe I'm also like that. If he's the first one, then maybe I'll get to be number two." But there has never been someone who has not died. We are all in the same boat, without exception. So we need to be skilled at dying.

Not just skilled for your own death, but also in your role as a doctor who deals with people who are in the process of dying. You need to be skilled at helping patients who are dying. People who are dying are filled with anxiety. There is a lot of physical pain, and there can be a lot of worry and fear. Some people are completely terrified. They are arriving at a time when they have to part with everything they have known: their friends, their families, their intimates, their children, their possessions. Everything. The thought of having to part with everything that they know can be almost too difficult to bear. While not wanting to part with any of it, they still depart. They still die. If they could bring some friends along, or some of the family, along with a few treasured possessions, then it wouldn't be so bad. But they cannot bring anything, not even their body. Everything is left behind. Everything is abandoned, discarded. That kind of feeling weighs acutely upon a patient's mind.

Of course patients might have an idea about what is going to happen after they die, according to their particular religion or belief, but honestly one really doesn't know for certain. So they tend to think "What is *really* going to happen?" no matter what kind of belief they already have. Right now we are not in the process of actually dying, so this is the time to prepare. This is the time to learn how to be ready, to make ourselves capable of dealing with the situation of dying when it finally arrives.

The part of you that knows and feels right now is your mind. When it comes time to die, that which knows and feels is the same mind.

And what continues to have experiences and go through whatever happens after death is also the same mind. It's not something other than that. Right now, while we are alive, we have a lot of freedom to choose what to do. Therefore, it makes sense to make the right choices. When we think about the prospect of our own death, and when we face other people's death, that experience is a like a teacher reminding us of the truth.

The fourth type of teacher is called the ultimate teacher of our innate nature. That teacher also has other names: *self-existing awareness, intrinsic mind, intrinsic wakefulness*, or the *unconditioned innate suchness*. That last one has a nice profound ring to it, doesn't it? But the purpose of these words is not just to *sound* profound. These words carry profound meaning; they refer to the basis for knowledge that can be brought into our own experience through training. This is of utmost importance. As a matter of fact, in a person's life, you could say that the most important goal would be to recognize and experience the unconditioned innate nature. Why? Because resting or remaining in a state of unconditioned innate nature liberates *any* emotional state. It frees you of the ignorant clinging to duality. As a matter of fact, there is no higher freedom that can be attained, or would be necessary to be attained.

Busy Westerners often feel that they don't have enough time to devote to spiritual practice, even if they think it might be of benefit. Like any other pursuit, it depends mainly on how much interest and importance you attach to it. Westerners are very developed at organizing and producing daily work. You can get a lot done in a day. If a person's normal daily activity seems interesting and rewarding, then spiritual practice may be only a kind of hobby. Even as a hobby, however, spiritual practice still has some benefit.

How much we choose to develop our own spiritual qualities is completely an individual matter. The Buddha once said that spiritual practice is something that is open to any person. Anyone is allowed to pursue spiritual practice, and there will be beneficial results for whoever chooses to do so, no matter who they are. The question then is how to best pursue spiritual practice. The answer is, in the ideal case, that you leave behind your ordinary daily life and focus one-pointedly on spiritual practice. The example for this is someone who goes into the mountains and stays in a cave and does little else besides spiritual training. In Tibet there was a very famous mountain yogi named Milarepa. You might enjoy reading his life story, called *The Life of Milarepa*.

The second way to pursue spiritual practice is to enter a monastic situation, in which everything is set up to allow individuals to develop their spiritual qualities. You can take the pledge of being either a monk or nun, and then there is a program that you would follow from morning to evening that involves study, meditation practice, discussion, and so forth.

The third way to pursue spiritual practice is the most difficult. That is to be a lay person. A lay person is defined as anyone actively involved in the tasks of daily living: a parent with children, a married person, a working person, or anyone who has many duties and tasks. In all these activities there are situations that provoke various emotional states: attachment, aggression, pride, jealousy, and other emotions. You live in a sea of emotions. If you are able, while being caught up in the reality of living your daily life, to still practice and attain accomplishment, you would actually be considered the best type of practitioner, because this is the most difficult path. The next best path would be to become a monastic type of person. The person who has the easiest time being a spiritual practitioner is someone who stays in a cave, off in the mountains, free of external distractions.

Within Buddhist philosophy, the practice of learning to recognize the ultimate teacher of our innate nature is considered the most important. In the beginning, becoming aware of our innate nature requires effort. It requires deliberately reminding ourselves. That's only in the beginning. Then, as one has more practice and training, reminding ourselves to recognize our own nature requires less and less effort. Our practice becomes smoother. As we become more and more stable in experiencing the compassionate emptiness of our innate nature, we notice that our involvement in blind emotions and negative actions becomes less and less. At the same time, we also notice that positive qualities—wisdom, compassion, and the capability to unfold and expand our consciousness more and more—begin to increase until we eventually reach what is called true and complete enlightenment.

17

Cultivating a Calm Mind

W HEN WE TRAIN IN MEDITATION, the first step is to allow our attention to be calm. Why? Because it is in the atmosphere of calm that intelligence and compassion naturally blossom. Like water clears when undisturbed, mind clears when undisturbed. During a human life, there is so much hope and fear, so much worry and anxiety, even in a single day. We experience all kinds of negative emotions—endlessly. We cannot always fulfill our expectations and ambitions. Just having unfulfilled desire in itself is painful. One way to pursue spiritual practice is to check which of our desires are realistic. How many of our ambitions can we honestly hope to achieve? It's good to have some pragmatic limits.

We may need permission, from time to time, to allow ourselves to relax, to not be so hard on ourselves—to simply be at ease and happy. We need to learn to be kind to ourselves. The more we let ourselves feel free and easy, the happier we are. The more stress we put on ourselves and constrict our way of being, the more uncomfortable we are. This is an obvious fact, one we are familiar with from our own experience.

If we want to be happy, we should learn what it takes to be happy. Feeling content is not primarily dependent upon external things. External things form the setting, but only the setting. The main thing is your mind. If you know how to allow your mind to be free and easy, then wherever you go, you'll be comfortable. Whomever you are with, it will be okay. On the other hand, if you are feeling frustrated, stressed, unhappy, or unfulfilled, wherever you go and whomever you are with, you'll still be uncomfortable.

For each and every one of us, the most important thing is our state of mind. That which feels joy or sorrow, pleasure or pain, is just our mind. But our mind doesn't have to simply react to things around us. It can be steered in different directions. You can direct yourself toward what is good, and by doing so, you get accustomed to positive thoughts. If you direct yourself toward being negative, that also can become a habit. If you allow yourself to become apathetic and not care much, you become insensitive and dull. The word *spiritual* refers to directing or steering our mind toward something good, something noble. Simply that. One of the most important factors in accomplishing that goal is to know how to let ourselves be completely at ease.

Many people try very hard to be physically healthy by engaging in various exercises and diets. A lot of energy is put into being physically well. Shouldn't we also be doing something to let our mind be healthy as well? Mind is more important than the body—the body is simply the mind's tool for doing things. When the mind thinks, "Get up and walk," the body gets up and walks. If the mind thinks, "Sit down," the body sits down.

Most of us lead very busy lives. The tasks that we are so busy carrying out usually have a purpose. Generally, we could say that this purpose is to ensure that what comes afterward is comfortable. In other words, our whole life is actually spent preparing for what comes next. This process carries some built-in anxiety because we are attached to a particular outcome. Wanting to make sure things go a certain way intrinsically creates hope and fear. Even a tiny worry about whether the future is going to be okay is always a little bit painful. If the aim of all our activity is to create well-being in our life, but the preparation consists of being ill at ease, when exactly do we accomplish our aim?

It is not necessary to be constantly worried about being well or happy. It's okay to relax. Of course we need to be attentive to how things are going. We can't completely ignore our responsibilities, but we don't have to be obsessively concerned either. We can take it easy some of the time. If it were *necessary* to worry and be anxious unremittingly in order to achieve our goals, then that would be fine. If it were *useful* to accomplish our aim, then we should do that. But actually we are just giving ourselves a hard time. I'm not saying you should be unconcerned with how your life is unfolding. There's just no need to be overly anxious.

If you want compassion and wisdom that is natural and uncontrived, it does not happen unless it arises from a calm state of mind. Training in being calm can be called meditation. You can also call it any other name you want. To be completely relaxed, you need to rest in a way that is beyond thinking, beyond concepts—and yet aware. This type of awareness can be termed *unconditioned suchness*. Resting in that state is the true relaxation. However, just relaxing and being calm is not the same as resting in unconditioned suchness. When we consciously try to relax and be calm, there is still the self-conscious sense of dwelling in a calm state. Notions are still present: "I am calm. I'm resting. I must be calm. Calm, calm, calm. Now I'm not calm anymore. I got up."

Suchness means our basic nature, something unconditioned that is present within each of us. When our attention is occupied with dualistic thinking, our basic nature is obscured, and the resultant state of mind is called *obscured suchness*. But the instant that this preoccupation with clinging to duality is allowed to subside and vanish, then that state of mind is called *unobscured suchness*.

Unconditioned suchness is already present as the nature of every sentient being, all of the time. All the trouble arises from simply not knowing that this is the case. It is quite likely that from time to time we have a moment when we are just present in our basic nature, but this experience is probably quite short. Since we aren't accustomed to recognizing this nature, we can't acknowledge it for what it is. Recognizing our basic nature has nothing to do with being religious or spiritual, or calling ourselves Buddhist. Since we are not in the habit of recognizing our basic nature, we simply can't nurture and extend these brief glimpses. As a result, we fail to prioritize what is really important. We just ignore our basic state and carry on with whatever we are doing. What is of truly vital importance is not recognized as such, and what is actually inconsequential we treat as being very important.

Our basic nature—whatever it truly is—becomes obvious to us the instant the state of mind that obscures our basic nature is allowed to vanish. That direct experience of our basic nature, even if it lasts only a moment, is called recognizing our natural state. This is true for any of us, no matter who we are. The terms *karma, obscurations,* and *disturbing emotions* describe states of mind in which our attention is clinging to duality. They all disappear the instant we recognize our unobscured suchness. What remains is profound compassion and wisdom.

There are many ways to relax and be calm. One could achieve a stupid, half-asleep state, like a bear in hibernation. Bears stay calm for many months in hibernation, but there is no awareness in that state. The best way is to be calm in a very present, lucid way. The calm feeling should be associated with an awake presence. That is the basis for the terms *thought-free wakefulness,* and *self-existing awareness,* which refer to a lucid state untainted by clinging. These terms come directly from a tradition within Tibetan Buddhism known as *dzogchen,* which is a particular form of practice that is an ultimate, direct way of training the mind in recognizing one's natural state.

Compassion and loving-kindness are the basic factors that create harmony and well-being for ourselves and others. Compassion is such a compelling quality that whenever a feeling of strong compassion comes into your mind, it clears away whatever negative emotions are present. They just fall away. At the same time compassion is of great benefit to those around you. When you experience pure and sincere compassion with an open and expansive frame of mind, at that very moment there is no longer any place for rivalry or anger. They have vanished. You may have experienced this yourself.

Let's say that your goal is to promote peace in the world. What is required is that everyone develops loving-kindness and compassion. There's no other way. We can't induce every other person in the world to immediately become more compassionate, so your primary responsibility is to make your own loving-kindness and compassion more open, more impartial. The purity of your compassion depends on your will, your motivation. One of the important points to keep in mind while striving to be kind is to expect less in return, to not hope for positive feedback or a reward. You need to avoid thinking, "I did a good deed, so they ought to treat me nicely in return. But they are not, so therefore I'm justified in feeling angry. I will certainly not bother to be kind to them next time." You want to avoid thinking like that.

As I've mentioned already, there are various levels of practice that we refer to with the word *meditation*. The first levels of meditation require some effort. Something is held in mind, and we apply some effort to keep something—a kind of focus—in our mind. This type of meditation has the effect of calming our mental processes, making our nature more gentle. The highest, most eminent form of practice is called *the great meditation of nonmeditation*. This practice is not a religion or a philosophy. It is not something new that was created by the Buddha. It is the original state—how our nature is already from the beginning. Nonmeditation refers to resting in *unconditioned suchness*. It is the quintessence of a calm mental state.

PRACTICAL ADVICE

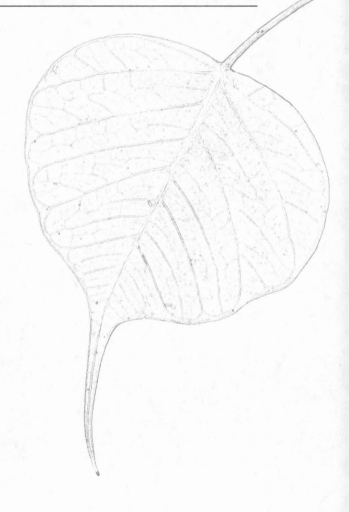

18

The Best Possible Care

W̲E̲ ̲A̲L̲L̲ ̲K̲N̲O̲W̲ that people suffer, in all the different variations that we have described. So the obvious question is what method could reduce suffering, or bring about freedom from suffering altogether, for ourselves and others? Although a certain amount of suffering seems to be built into our lives, it is a fact that, the more we can loosen up the rigid tendency to hold onto things, the less suffering and pain we will experience in any situation. Being able to let go even helps when you are experiencing physical pain—the pain can feel less severe. On the other hand, even a little physical pain can feel unbearable if we are mentally unprepared to deal with it. The same is true for emotional stresses.

When we are faced with an incident that we believe is unpleasant, we focus our whole attention on it. But if, soon after that, something even more unpleasant happens, we totally forget the previous situation—it suddenly seems unimportant. At that moment, the attachment to the previous situation vanishes, and along with it the pain that it was causing us. If we could develop the ability to completely release the tendency to hold something firmly in our minds, to fixate, then any type of suffering could be overcome. Even if we aren't able to completely get rid of suffering immediately, if we can just loosen its hold a little bit, we'll find that suffering decreases correspondingly.

Now it happens that people fall ill. Young people can fall ill, and also old people. When an older person falls ill, it may become clear at some point that the illness is terminal, and the person dies. Such a death may feel kind of acceptable, either because the person reached such an advanced age that it feels natural to die at that point, or the disease became so severe and prolonged that death appears to be a relief. When death comes at an advanced age, it doesn't seem like such a disaster. It appears to involve less suffering.

However, we must be careful when we start to think about death at an old age in this way. If we think that it is normal for older people to become sick and die, then we may start to think, "Okay, now this person is old and has become sick. There's no hope." This may lead to less care. Due to feeling that there is no point in trying to cure the patient because they are so old anyway, we may just put the person away from view. We might just check once in a while to see if they are still alive. Old age becomes an excuse for not putting as much effort into the care of that person. It's painful to think about older people lying alone and frightened as the end of their life draws near.

At the same time, if a young person falls seriously ill, that person gets a lot of attention. Why is that? It may be that some people think about the human body the way some people feel about cars. When you have an expensive new car, you feel that any damage must be fixed. If you have an old car, you are not concerned about small scratches or even more major damage. If the car stops running, you just throw it away. If you are not careful, society may mistake the human body for a piece of machinery. I'm joking, of course, but there is some truth in the joke.

Whether the person we are caring for is an infant, a child, a teenager, an adult, or someone in advanced age, we should always try our best to give the best possible care. I'm not talking just about medical help that can cure, or surgery if that is necessary. I'm talking about taking care of the person's well-being, and giving tender, loving care—

being as kind and considerate as possible and attending to every need no matter what the age. Look at them with kind eyes and hold their hand with kindness. Console them by speaking in an appropriate way. The appropriateness of what you say will vary from individual to individual. You may say something that is true but sounds awful to an ailing patient. That's not very helpful. Even when you can't console with words or do some medical procedure that helps, just showing a kind face is an effective way to ease a patient's mind.

This is especially important for the doctor or the medical practitioner who is most responsible for the person's care. The doctor must avoid showing a fear of coming too close, or revealing by the look on his or her face the feeling of "I've given up on you." You don't want to give the impression of being uncomfortable being around the patient because you feel that you have nothing to offer or that there is no hope. From the point of view of the patient, who is in a very sensitive state, just seeing someone look at them like that can be overwhelmingly painful.

When we think about what it means to give the best possible care, we should think about how patients react in painful and frightening situations, and use all of our wisdom and compassion to help relieve their suffering.

19

Coping with Difficult Patients and Situations

I T IS ALWAYS EASIER to be kind to a person that you know and care about. This is true whether you are a medical professional, a school teacher, a professor, or a spiritual teacher, such as a lama. We always feel that it is easier to help someone who listens to what we say and responds intelligently. We may actually experience delight or pleasure when we help someone we like and who appreciates our actions. Doctors feel good when they are able to take care of a cooperative patient, one who understands what you tell him or her and follows directions. When the patient behaves like a decent human being, you are better able to utilize your skills. This is the kind of patient who respects your abilities and is able to express gratitude. The moment you walk in the door, they smile and are happy to see you.

What happens when we are faced with the opposite kind of patient? The moment you walk in the door, they get unhappy. Whatever advice you give them, they ignore it. They may be short-tempered and irritable, and lash out verbally. They may express anger at their treatment and the doctor. They want to get better, but they feel they are not getting better fast enough. They refuse to listen to explanations.

Frankly speaking, it's not easy to deal with people like that. It's as if there is a barrier to giving good care. Whether this kind of patient produces a lot of anger and resentment in a doctor or nurse varies from caregiver to caregiver. Some doctors or nurses might feel very angry and deeply resentful. Others might feel a moderate amount of resentment, and a few may be only slightly upset by their encounter. However, it is likely that everyone experiences at least some kind of negative reaction toward a difficult patient. If you discover that you feel no resentment or resistance at all in dealing with such a person, then you can take it as a sure sign that you have already achieved very good results in training in compassion!

Whenever you encounter a person who is irritable, aggressive, or uncooperative, you can view this as a special opportunity to generate compassion. The fact that the patient is acting this way means that the person is feeling disturbed, not at ease. They are not mentally disturbed in the sense of being insane, but they simply can't handle what they are going through. That's why they are irritable.

There is always a reason why a person gets angry. For example, in Tibet we recognize a specific type of anger that comes from being hungry. In the Tibetan language there is a word that translates as "hungry anger." I don't believe there is a specific word for that feeling in English. Children seem to have "hungry anger" often—perhaps every day. In any case, if we are honest with ourselves, we also get irritable in response to different kinds of stress. Not just when we are hungry, but also when we get tired.

If we get irritable just from being hungry or tired, it seems unavoidable that we will feel irritable when we are ill. When a person is irritable due to feeling ill, they are not necessarily in control of their emotional state. Ironically, they often focus their anger on the person they rely on the most. They become annoyed with their parents, their friends, or their spouse. Sometimes the ill person has the feeling that they have a right to be served by whoever is near them, and if that person doesn't respond fast enough, they become even more upset.

People who are ill find themselves dependent on others for help. In most cases, the patient must place their trust in a doctor, hoping the doctor will be able to make them better. There are many different kinds of diseases, some of which may feel nearly unbearable. This is especially true for diseases that have no cure.

If the doctor says, "I'm sorry, there's nothing that can be done to cure your illness," the patient will feel some resentment. Even if the disease *is* impossible to cure, and the doctor is simply being honest, the patient may still get angry. It's not what the patient wants to hear. When a patient is seriously ill, it can be very difficult to endure the pain and discomfort. Just trying to cope with the pain from moment to moment can lead to a feeling of anguish and hopelessness. The patient feels that there has to be *some* solution to his or her suffering. When that doesn't happen, the patient gets angry, and the anger may be directed toward the doctor. They may say, "I hate the doctor. He's supposed to cure me, so why doesn't he?" It may look this way from the patient's point of view because the patient is upset. When someone is feeling extremely agitated or aggressive, they may say whatever comes into their mind without thinking first.

I would like to introduce an approach to dealing with patients who may feel that they can't take it anymore, who are aggressive, irritable, or in pain. Although we should, of course, be compassionate toward everyone who is ill, we should be *especially* compassionate toward the irritable, unpleasant patient—someone who does *not* appreciate you, someone who, without any obvious reason, gets angry. What can we do under those circumstances to remain compassionate? We need to maintain a sense of tolerance, for when you lose your tolerance, it's hard to be compassionate. However, if you are willing to bear the patient's irritation, it's much easier to be compassionate, to have patience toward their behavior.

Patience is like an armor, and the stronger your compassion, the stronger the armor. This is an intelligent way to approach compassion.

In other words, there is some insight associated with your compassionate state of mind. When insight is present, you don't become weary or discouraged. Your compassion needs to be suffused with this intelligent quality of seeing clearly. Otherwise, when you are confronted with people who don't want to listen to you, even when you've tried your best to be kind and caring, you may feel discouraged. You may think, "Why should I bother? I give up. They don't listen to what I say."

Physical suffering is one thing. But compared to physical suffering, mental suffering can be even worse, almost impossible to bear. For example, you may encounter patients who are not really physically ill, but in their own mind are experiencing pain and anguish that seems unbearable to them. From your point of view, you may feel that they are irrational, that they should just come to their senses. This is when you may feel weary and lose patience.

When this happens you must once again put on your armor of patience. Again and again. Try to be as compassionate as possible. However, despite all of your efforts, you may come a point at which you feel that you have truly tried your best—that to keep pushing would put you beyond your limit. Pushing yourself past that point will only make you irritable and angry, and there is no benefit in that because those emotions don't help the patient or yourself. Therefore it's necessary to keep a balance, to learn when to draw the line. Otherwise, even though you have tried so hard, been so patient, and used your sense of perseverance and strength to the utmost, things could turn out badly. By pushing yourself too far, you annoy the patient and get fed up yourself. You go home and wake up the next morning feeling, "What's the use?" You begin to feel discouraged. A self-defeating attitude begins to crop up, and that's a danger.

Whether we are doing a normal kind of job or have spiritual responsibilities, we always need to keep a sense of balance. Even when pouring a glass of water we need to achieve the right balance. If we pour too much the glass overflows. If we pour too little there's not enough to drink. If your aim is bad the water spills. In whatever we do, whether it is cooking a full meal or just making tea or coffee, it requires the right measure. If we use too many coffee grounds, the coffee will taste bad. If we don't use enough grounds, the coffee will be too weak. It also depends on individual taste. If we put too much milk in the coffee some people won't like it. Some people want their coffee black. Some want sugar only, while some want milk and sugar.

We need that sense of the appropriate measure, a sense of balance. But what we consider the right measure is not the same for everyone. Everyone has their own limits, their own level of how much they can do and how much they need. If we know our limits, if we know our boundaries, that's called being wise. If we don't know our own limits and boundaries, we can't call that wise. It's called being thickheaded. A thick-headed person doesn't know his or her own boundaries. Such a person needs to be told by a superior, "Now stay put, now move, now stop." This is necessary when a person doesn't know his or her own limits and boundaries.

On the other hand, a wise person is someone who has evaluated his or herself and is able to achieve a balanced quality of being. Someone who understands the intentions and needs of others. For example, at a dinner party when the host says, "Please stay longer," you may perceive that it's just a superficial request, and say, "That's very kind of you, but I have to leave now." You know not to overstay your welcome. That's an example of being wise.

There are many levels of limitations and boundaries. There is an obvious level, an inner level, and a very subtle level as well. To learn to understand your boundaries and limitations is wise. When it comes to medication, it has to be given in the right dose at the right times. The amount and type of medicine needs to be chosen and measured very carefully. If you give too much, there's a danger, and if you give too little, there is no effect. That holds true for many things. Giving medication is an example, but there a lot of things like that.

There is a balance that is necessary in all of our activities: how much we move around, how we much we sit, how much we speak, how long we sleep. For all of these activities there is some right measure, some balance to be achieved. Eating too much is not good. It can be a great burden to eat so much that you become grossly overweight. Choosing not to eat to such an extent that you become painfully thin is also not good. When you choose the right measure in between, it feels very comfortable.

Compassion has incredible qualities. However, we need to appreciate when we have done all that we can do. We need to develop the confidence that we have tried our best. We need to recognize when we have given our best care, and have been willing to be kind. In that way, we begin to appreciate our abilities as healers. Instead of feeling depressed, discouraged, and tired, we can be bolstered by our own sense of confidence: "I know that I have sincerely tried my best. I've tried to care for this person as much as I can, and to be kind. I should feel good about the effort that I've made." That's one point.

At the same time, however, we want to avoid drawing a line too soon with the thought, "I've had enough." We need to be willing to continue. In addition to recognizing that you have tried your best, you still need to remain open to what else can be done. You need to think, "I feel that I have already done my best, and yet there must be something left to try." It is possible that there is still something that can be tried that you haven't yet considered. If we think that way, we may be able to find someone else who can help with the situation. I'm not talking about trying to run away from the situation or pass the buck. I'm talking about the willingness to bring in other people with insights and capacity that could be helpful in addition to one's own.

There is a kind of purity associated with this type of compassion. A purity that comes from trying to find the most effective care. It is probably impossible for a doctor to be completely unkind without even a shred of compassion. But it is possible for a doctor to become less sensitive to the suffering that he or she has to deal with. If there are too many patients in a day, too many serious problems, a doctor can begin to feel that this kind of suffering is just routine, and stop caring about the individual people who are ill. When we have seen too much suffering, suffering people no longer affect us in the same way.

When you first start training as a doctor, you are more sensitive to the suffering of others. When you see patients in pain for the first time, you are more aware of their suffering. As you start to see more and more patients, you become a little less sensitive. Suffering begins to seem routine. That acute sense of caring about how the patient feels wears off as time passes. Using intelligent compassion can prevent becoming hardened to the patient's worries. Compassion allows you to continue to want to relieve their suffering, and intelligence can help you understand where their suffering is actually coming from. This can help you feel less overwhelmed and exhausted when facing people who are suffering and irritable.

We shouldn't lose sight of the main point, that it is not a matter of creating compassion, but a process of just allowing it to occur. Just like water is wet, or a flame is hot, our basic nature is inherently compassionate. Developing our compassion is a matter of allowing it to grow forth, to cultivate something already present within us.

In order to be able to apply compassion wisely, we need to remind ourselves about the causes of suffering. Suffering is related to how attached a person is to the pain and discomfort that they are experiencing. The more a person focuses on the pain and discomfort, the deeper the suffering. If there is only a medium level of attachment or clinging, the pain is only that much. For someone who is able to be totally unattached, there is no sense of suffering, even if their body is experiencing the causes of pain.

The root cause of suffering, and of all negative emotions, is cling-ing. Clinging means "to hold in mind." So how can we be completely free from "holding in mind" without simply replacing one thought with another? This is where we utilize the concept that I mentioned earlier of learning to recognize our innate suchness—our basic awareness beyond thought. It is a very important point. Not only does recogniz-ing our basic nature help relieve suffering, it allows the qualities of compassion and wisdom to grow and stabilize. Our armor of patience grows thicker, and our ability to intelligently find solutions becomes easier. We will no longer be so worn out by difficult patients.

Sometimes it is not the patient that is difficult, but the situation itself. It can feel overwhelming for the caregiver not to be able to save a patient's life. The doctor or the nurse who is involved in treating someone should try their best, with their physical actions, their words, and their attitude. After having tried one's best, if the patient doesn't get better, or dies, then it is not a result of the fact that you didn't offer what you could. It's okay to still feel sad about it—you can even take the feeling of sadness as a good sign. Why? It means that you truly have loving-kindness—you care. You are not a machine. However, to keep doubting yourself and wishing that you could have done more, over and over, is of no use. It's not a healthy attitude.

The best way to avoid doubt and regret is to realize that we need to do our best when actually dealing with the patient. We need to utilize our body, speech, and mind, and to seek help when we need it. Then if our efforts fail to make the situation better, it isn't because we didn't *try* to help, it's because we *couldn't* help. You need to distinguish between these two words. If you could have done something more and didn't, that is different. If you only tried half as hard as you could, that's very different from not being able to heal somebody. Even if you gave 80 to 90 percent, there is the possibility of feeling regret. If you apply yourself 100 percent for the patient's benefit and the person doesn't keep living, then it is not because you didn't do what you could, it's because you couldn't.

Being incapable of saving people is the nature of things. That fact cannot be changed. When we are unable to save someone, it's okay to feel sad, but we can also have a sense of rejoicing. We feel sad because we were not able to change the outcome, but we can rejoice in knowing that we did our best. One hundred percent effort. The result is often a bittersweet feeling, because it's true that you were incapable of saving that person. You cannot save everyone all the time, but at the same time you can feel good about yourself because you did your best.

One of the really difficult questions that arises in a doctor or nurse's life is how to help comfort a child who is dying, and how to help the parents of the child. It is our human nature to view dying as more easy to accept if someone first becomes old before they die. This feels easier to us. If someone is young and healthy and then becomes sick and dies we feel more sad, more hurt. We ask ourselves, "Why does a child die? Why couldn't they become old before they died?" There are two possible replies. One is that they just got a bad disease—it's a random accident, just bad luck. The spiritual practitioner, however, will say it's karma—the result of cause and effect. Either way, it's a bad situation. To become sick and die is very bad.

Now the question is how to respond to this situation. Just being worried and sad, feeling helpless and hopeless, will not help yourself and will definitely not help the child who is dying. It's at these moments that we need to be strong. The parents also need to be strong. They need to offer their full attention, care, and love from their side. It's good if they can consult more than one doctor, in order to feel that they have done all that they can do. This is a very good tradition in America, a second opinion. If the parents do the best they can, just as we described for the doctor, the parents will also end up with the same bittersweet feeling. They couldn't save their child, but it's not because they didn't try their best. It's because it couldn't be helped. That's a different feeling. That's very important. Couldn't and didn't. If you didn't do all that you could, then there is cause for regret. That can be hard to shake. If it happens that the child dies and it couldn't be helped, of course one feels regret, but it's not reasonable to blame yourself. It's important to make this distinction.

20

Easing the Process of Dying

ONE OF THE THINGS that makes medical practitioners most uncomfortable is trying to help someone who is dying. The topic of death and dying is part of the larger theme of impermanence. Before we talk specifically about dying, it is important to recall our discussion about impermanence. We need to understand deeply, not just intellectually, that whatever is formed or produced does not last. Once we recognize and accept the fact of impermanence, it is much easier to accommodate whatever happens—pleasure, pain, joy, or sorrow. Why? Because we can understand that they all pass.

Let's say that you have not accepted the fact that things are impermanent. Then, when something awful happens, you feel you can't stand it. It can be unbearable. The fact that everything formed is impermanent is not just some idea the Buddha had. It's a fact that each and every one of us can observe for ourselves if we take the time to think about it. There are a lot of ways to describe the impermanence of all things, but there are four major points worth mentioning.

1. *Building ends in crumbling.* Whatever has been constructed, made, produced, or created will all fall apart in the end, sooner or later. It's only a matter of time.

2. *Gathering ends in depletion.* No matter how much we bring together, it runs out at some point. It's impossible for that not to be so.

Name, power, position, money, material—whatever we gain, whatever we have, gets used up. It vanishes.

3. *Meeting ends in parting.* There is temporary parting from the ones we love, and there is permanent separation. All meeting ends in separation. There is no exception, no escape from that reality.

4. *Birth ends in death.* No one ever born has escaped death. In the past it never happened, right now it's impossible, and in the future it will never happen either. Why? Because everything formed is by nature impermanent.

I'm not referring just to living things. Everything is impermanent—whatever we see, hear, smell, taste, and touch. Whatever comes into existence does so for a while and then perishes. Not only do things change in the long run, they change every instant. These tiny changes are not visible with the naked eye. I once saw a movie taken through a microscope. Even when everything on the microscope was completely still, the particles under the lens were constantly shaking.

Impermanence is a fact, and it's sensible to view things as they really are. There's a definite benefit from accepting that all things pass. It helps us be more balanced and healthy. Normally, the tendency to hold on strongly to things as being real, permanent, and lasting creates enormous tension when those things prove to be otherwise. Whenever something good or pleasant happens, we feel sad when it ends. Whenever something awful takes place, we naturally become unhappy. However, when we realize that all these events are impermanent, good or bad, it allows us to tolerate change more easily, and we become more resilient.

While most of us intellectually recognize this impermanent nature of things, we usually don't spend much time thinking about it. When we hear about impermanence, it is helpful to reflect on what it means, to come to grips with its reality. Through such reflection, we can begin to pay more attention to our experiences in light of impermanence, and confirm for ourselves, on a deep level, that things do undergo constant change.

The time spent contemplating and studying impermanence prepares us to accept that the body dies. It's just a natural consequence of being alive. While you are alive, it is important to learn how to live in such a way that you can be at ease with whatever happens. When dying, it's important to learn how to die in a way that is not so burdened by anxiety, fear, or pain—to learn how to die without dread.

Buddhist teachers emphasize the concept of "impermanence" a great deal, with good reason. If you spend time contemplating the fact of impermanence, when it comes time to face your own death it is easier for someone to help remind you. They might say, "All things must pass—nothing lasts." And you will think, "Yes, that's true." Because you have already made yourself familiar with this fact, it becomes easier to admit it, to take it to heart, and to relax a little bit. Without reflecting on impermanence and taking it to heart, people can be overly attached to things and people as being permanent in their lives. Then, when something goes wrong, they have a very difficult time accepting it. They may panic and keep asking, "Why? Why is this happening to me?" Why not? Everything is impermanent. Impermanence is a great teacher.

How can we use this knowledge in comforting someone who is dying, or the family of that person? While there is still a chance to cure the present illness, we should of course encourage them to try to get better, to keep hope. However, once it has become completely clear that there is no chance of recovery and death is inevitable, we can try to help them not fight it so much, not let it be such a burden. We can try our best to help them accept that dying is the natural course of things—that there is an end. This is how you can help any dying person or family member.

However, we must not use the fact that someone is dying to avoid taking very good physical care of them. We need to treat them very nicely, very gently. We need to hold their hand, speak nicely, and help them relax. We can tell them, "Don't worry. What is happening to you is natural, just take it easy. Whatever you need to make you more comfortable, we will try to do it."

Accepting that death is natural and inevitable may not initially feel comforting to some patients who have not spent time thinking about impermanence. Most people who are dying are very attached to their family, to material things, or to something else that they can't take with them. We need to encourage them to let go, because it is the attachments that create so much stress and fear. Whoever is close to the person, whoever has their trust, should offer gentle care and encourage the person to relax and let go. Particularly if you are dealing with someone who is not a spiritual practitioner, agonizing fear and pain may arise at the thought of parting from their family and their belongings. To help them reduce their clinging, you can gently say, "What is the use of holding on now? It will only cause yourself more pain. It's okay to let go." This is a conventional way of trying to comfort people who are dying.

If the person who is dying is a spiritual person, it's a somewhat different matter. The spiritual person may believe that although the body dies, the mind or spirit does not. If you believe that the mind carries on after death, the problem of attachment is viewed differently. From this point of view, attachment is not only a problem while you are about to die, but it can remain a problem at the moment of death and beyond. Therefore, it is even more crucial to try to let go of all of your attachments before you die.

People can be attached to many different things. The strongest attachments are usually toward other people, but you can also be attached to a particular object, some property, or even a place with beautiful scenery. There are so many things that you could be very fond of and not want to part with. The dying person is rarely happy to lose everything that he or she knows and cares about. The dying person would like to be able to bring along loved ones, cherished possessions, and so forth, but he or she does not have the power to do so. It is not possible to bring anything. Even though they don't want to, they still have to lose it all.

The key point, therefore, is to let go—to let go of all you hold dear. If you are attached to property, possessions, and so forth, it's a good idea to give them away before you die, either to your family or to a good cause. In this way, you can begin to part with it in your mind and to feel more free. Of course you don't want to leave your parents, brothers, sisters, children, and spouse behind. But if you know you have to leave, it's important to part with them on good terms—to wish them well. Relatives and friends should also be encouraged to part with the dying person by expressing good wishes. They should avoid holding on tightly and saying, "Don't leave, don't leave," over and over again. That kind of display is an obstacle at the point when parting is inevitable. It's far better to let go, allowing the person to die peacefully after having given up attachments. Cutting the ties of attachment benefits any person, whether they are spiritual or not.

If the dying person is a spiritual practitioner who has received some specific instructions during his or her life, there is something more that they can do. They can utilize the practice called the *ejection of consciousness*. In the Tibetan language this is called *powa*, and it is basically a technique for ensuring the best trajectory for the mind as it leaves this body and begins its journey to the next.

It is also important, if the dying person knows how, to rest the mind in equanimity and to pass away in that state. The most important thing for a dying person is to be emotionally undisturbed—to be at peace. In general, the family and the people caring for the dying person should make it a priority not to disturb the dying person emotionally. Their focus should be to help the person relax, be at ease, and at peace. Dying at peace is dying skillfully.

When I am called to the bedside of someone who is dying, I try to take the following approach. First of all, I try to find out what that person trusts in. What is their belief? Then I can understand what is positive and good in their life, what gives their life meaning. If they are a spiritual practitioner, I try to remind them of their particular practice. I try to refresh their memory about what they have been taught and what they have practiced.

There have been different approaches in regard to how much information to give a person who is seriously ill with what may prove to be a fatal illness. On the one hand, it may seem beneficial to tell a dying person what you think is the truth about their illness, but on the other hand, it may be very painful and difficult for the patient to accept. In recent years in the West, doctors are more comfortable telling what they think is the truth. If the disease is not curable, they feel compelled to tell the patient what they think, otherwise they feel like they are lying. In the East, the doctors will often tell a lie—purposely hide the truth. Why does the doctor lie in this instance? Is this based on bad motivation or good motivation? It could very well be good motivation. In what circumstance would we call it good? Many doctors in the East believe that the mind has power. Instead of stressing the incurable nature of their disease, the doctor might say, "You will be okay. If you try hard and keep wishing for health, you might survive. Even in cases where the disease is quite advanced, there are some cases in which people have survived. Don't give up hope." Talking like this can give the patient power to deal with their illness. When a serious disease like cancer is first diagnosed, the doctor may know some statistics that make the outlook very bleak, but there is a choice at that point about how to share that information with the patient.

Scientific studies in the West have demonstrated that patients can have some control over their illness through the power of their mind. This is also compatible with Buddhist belief. As a result of hearing a positive presentation of their situation, a sick person might think, "The doctor told me that I might be okay. So I will eat good food, take the medicine, and get some exercise. I will become stronger." They feel happier because they have some hope. They feel that they have a chance. If you say instead, "Sorry, there's no hope," then the patient thinks, "Why should I even bother to take the medicine?" At that point the patient only experiences fear, and gives up hope. That may decrease their ability to fight the disease.

I think it is best to try to find a middle way somewhere in between these extremes. Honesty is of course desirable. However, sometimes attempting to be too honest is not really being honest. For example, if you say, "I think your disease is incurable," that may reflect what you truly think at the time. But what happens if that person later recovers? Does that mean you lied? If the disease is really bad, you could say, "Your disease is not an easy disease to cure, but we need to try. We both need to have some hope. We'll try our best, and you can try your best." The idea is to try to avoid cutting off all hope.

Once the situation is unavoidably hopeless, and the person is facing death, we can change our approach. We then need to address the problem of the best way to relieve their suffering. These days, doctors have available very strong drugs that can relieve the pain associated with dying. These drugs can be effective, but they can also cloud the patient's mind. Since we have been talking about the mental state one should try to have when one is dying, it may be confusing as to how to administer these drugs in a particular situation.

As a healing professional, you will need to use your own wisdom. There is no fixed answer for this, because you need to evaluate each situation individually. What kind of person is the patient? How much of a spiritual practitioner—a true practitioner—is the person? How much pain can that person actually deal with without negatively affecting their state of mind? You need to determine what is most appropriate, where to draw the line. It would be best if some degree of awareness is preserved, instead of making the person completely oblivious. At the same time, you don't want to force the person to suffer needlessly. You need to seek some kind of balance between those two choices. That's an individual judgement that the doctor has to make.

I've heard from people who work with dying patients that it sometimes seems as if the religious beliefs of the patient are actually increasing fear at the end of life rather than offering comfort. This can be an awkward situation for the doctor or nurse. In the Buddhist tradition, when someone approaches death, there's one quality that is extremely important, and that is to have absolved one's self—literally. It doesn't matter to whom you have said sorry, or who you imagine that you express your apology to. The most important thing is that you feel afterward that you have actually let go of whatever you may feel that you have done wrong in thought, word, or deed. You admit what you have done wrong, apologize sincerely, and then imagine that it's all purified, gone, forgiven. You need to completely let go of those thoughts so that they no longer burden you. It makes you feel very carefree—unburdened, clear, and calm.

The doctor or nurse can encourage the person to let go of burdensome feelings and worries. You can tell them that it is possible to let go: "Yes you can. You can let it go." But you can't let go for them. They have to let go themselves. Your duty is to just assist to the best of our ability. As you gently encourage them to let go of all those feelings and worries, you can try to look at them with a kind face and focus all of your kindness and attention on them. Even if they are not able to give up 100 percent of their fears and worries, they may be able to let go of

20 or 30 percent. If they are intelligent and open-minded, they may be able to let go of 90 percent. But even 10 to 20 percent will help. We can try to help them feel at ease, to let go of their fear of punishment. We can try to help them release all of the attachments that are causing them pain. We can help them die at peace—skillfully.

21

The True Meaning of
Death with Dignity

I've ALREADY TALKED about how you can help a person die more peacefully. However, it is possible to develop even more skill in dying, such that you could actually approach your death with a positive attitude. If you are a spiritual practitioner, with experience in meditation, it is possible to view the death process as something to be experienced in a conscious way. Being able to die consciously and without fear provides a very favorable circumstance for quick progress on the path to enlightenment. Certain stages of spiritual realization that would ordinarily take a long time can be covered very rapidly at that point. The practitioner can be guided through the various stages of dying by a teacher or close spiritual friend, and that person can remind you that what you are experiencing are normal stages of the death process. Tibetan Buddhism teaches that as the physical body begins to disintegrate, the forces of the five elements each releases its grip on consciousness accompanied by a certain sign. A spiritual friend can point out what stage you are experiencing, and because you have studied and trained yourself in dying, you can accept and appreciate that.

In the teachings on Vajrayana, the esoteric path of Tibetan Buddhism, there is a description of four *bardos,* or transition periods in one's existence. The first bardo begins the moment you leave your mother's womb. You take your first breaths, you grow, and then, at some point near the end of this life, the circumstances are such that you know for sure that you will die. This could be due to a disease or an accident, but in any case, you recognize the end is near. The stretch of time from your first breath to the moment at which you know that dying has begun is called the *bardo of birth and living*. It's interesting to note that when a mother gives birth to a child, the first thing the child does is cry, and at the time of death, too, people cry. The moment the baby first comes out of the mother's womb, tears come, and if you look closely as people expire, there are also tears. It could be interesting to investigate why. Of course it is reasonable to cry at death, but why not laugh when taking birth?

The next bardo is the *bardo of dying*. It begins the moment at which the body will definitely not recover and survive, and it lasts until the last breath is exhaled. This bardo is accompanied by certain subjective experiences. In Buddhist tradition these experiences are explained as the dissolution of the elements. These dissolution experiences include a feeling of heaviness, feeling cold, and drying up of the mouth and nostrils. These are part of the specific signs that death is near. Finally, outer breathing, our normal respiration, is distinguished from inner breathing, which is more like circulation of energy. First the outer breathing stops, then the inner circulation of energy also stops. Some specific experiences are said to take place at that moment, and they end in a lapse of consciousness, called "fainting." Following fainting, there is a re-awakening from that state of oblivion.

The next bardo is the *luminous bardo of our innate nature*. In this stage, our innate nature—the basic nature of mind—is totally unobscured for a short while. We can glimpse our basic nature of mind at that moment. This is the same for every sentient being. This quality of mind, this "luminous wakefulness," is revealed to us at that moment—but it may be only a brief glimpse. The tendency to cling to duality is poised to reassert itself, and for most of us, it immediately moves in and obscures this experience of our basic nature.

Let's say, however, that the dying person was someone who, during his or her lifetime, was not only introduced to the basic nature of mind, but also trained in recognizing it and achieved some degree of stability. When such a person arrives at the bardo of the innate nature, he or she will already be familiar with remaining in that state of mind. At that point they may experience "the meeting between the mother and child luminous wakefulness," or the recognition of their own buddha nature in the same spontaneous way that a child recognizes its own mother. In that moment there is an opportunity to become fully liberated.

If you have some training in sustaining the nondual original mind, what we have also called *unconditioned suchness,* then the opportunity to be liberated exists immediately after awakening from the faint that occurs at the moment of death. If you have the ability to remain stable in recognizing luminous wakefulness, you can be liberated. Otherwise, confusion reasserts itself. If that happens, there is no other choice than the fourth bardo, the *karmic bardo of becoming.* "Becoming" here means seeking rebirth. That is why when a spiritual practitioner draws near the moment of death, it is extremely important to remember these instructions, and to remember the spiritual teacher. If you remember your spiritual teacher, you will immediately remember what you have been told to do at this point. If you can remember that, there is immense benefit.

In the karmic bardo of becoming, you are seeking a new rebirth. According to the Buddhist view, consciousness is something that continues, it doesn't just vanish. Therefore there is the possibility to take rebirth. The karmic bardo of becoming is generally said to last forty-nine days. During the first half of these forty-nine days, you may not yet have figured out that you have died. You move around, and the memories and impressions and so forth look very much like what you were used to when you were alive. You try to connect with past acquaintances and loved ones, but it is no longer possible. At some point you find out that you have died, and you begin to move toward your new life. Increasingly, the scenery and impressions begin to look like the place where you will next take rebirth.

What kind of body do you have in that bardo state? It's said to be a mental body, made out of habitual tendencies—our habits of thinking. Your body is very similar to the kind of body you run around in while dreaming. During a dream, your physical body remains lying in your bed, but your dream body moves around, doing all sorts of things. It feels as if you have a body, but you don't. That is the same type of body that the mind has while moving around in this bardo. Therefore, you may not immediately realize that you have passed away. The mental body is endowed with certain powers. All the five senses are intact, but you can move through solid matter in an instant. The moment you think of being somewhere—you are suddenly there. Why? Because it is not a physical body, it's just made of thoughts—it's a mental projection. It is this very ability to move around instantly that causes the person to suddenly realize, "I didn't used to be able to do this. Maybe I'm dead." That realization can be terribly frightening and can induce a real sense of panic.

Because of the tendency for the person in this bardo to panic, it is considered very important, in the Buddhist tradition, to perform good deeds and make good wishes on behalf of the dead person during the forty-nine days following death. All those connected with the dead person are encouraged to do that. Such methods are said to alleviate the bardo being's anguish and fear of being disembodied, and it may even help them to not suffer at all, or at least reduce the suffering, and help inspire them to seek a good rebirth, one conducive to further spiritual development.

The moment of experiencing the luminous bardo of our innate nature is like a fork in the road. We have an opportunity to go either one way or the other—either be liberated or continue to be confused. Therefore, true dignity in the face of death derives from the confidence that you have gained from your personal spiritual practice. You are familiar with your basic nature, and you know that it is possible to be liberated. That is the source of true dignity. A semblance of dignity comes from being undisturbed by worry, anxiety, and other self-oriented emotions at the time of death. We can achieve that sense of dignity from having trained in being calm and unattached to the fleeting things of this life.

The ability to die in a dignified manner has everything to do with how we spend our life. We can't all of a sudden notice that our time to die is coming near and try to make ourselves feel a certain way—at that point it's too late. We need to prepare ourselves while we have time, which means while we are still alive, before we actually begin to die. Dignity refers to a sense of self-respect, appreciation, and confidence. If we can carry that feeling through the dying process, that is the true meaning of death with dignity.

22

Tibetan Medicine

ALTHOUGH WE HAVE FOCUSED mainly on Western medicine in this book, it may be worthwhile to finish with a brief description of Tibetan medicine. You might benefit by knowing how Tibetan doctors incorporate some of the principles and training that we have been discussing.

In the Tibetan tradition, medicine is taught as one of the five sciences, or topics of knowledge, in centers for Buddhist training. The five sciences include healing (the practice of medicine), language, craftsmanship, logic, and inner science (spiritual practice and understanding). Tibetan medicine dates back over 2,500 years. Textbooks on how to diagnose and treat disease were available in Tibet long before Buddhist teachings were introduced in the eighth century. When Buddhism arrived in Tibet, this traditional medicine became much more standardized. The basis and practice of Tibetan medicine are explained and defined in authoritative scriptures, which have not yet been fully translated into English.

Within the Tibetan medical system there are three basic types of disease. The first type is called "physical disorder." The second type is translated as "bad energy," or "evil influence." The third type is called "emotional disorder."

The physical disorders are due to three primary factors, called wind, gall, and phlegm, and the combinations of these factors.* The combinations of imbalances have been categorized, and give rise to 404 primary types of illness. There are also subsidiary types of illness, so many as to be almost countless.

Disease due to evil influence is explained in a different way than physical illness. If someone with a scientific mind reads about something called "evil influence," they may laugh and simply dismiss the concept. But some readers with open minds might say, "I wonder what he actually means by that?" There are three types of evil influence: male influence, female influence, and neutral influence. If we look at the relationship between an ill person's way of perceiving and what is referred to as evil influence, it can be very revealing.

The diagnosis of evil influence is given in some cases with symptoms that Western doctors might diagnose as schizophrenia, intense paranoia, or hysteria. In those kinds of mental states, the patient may see what is not present or hear voices other people do not. In the West these are called "delusional states." Where do these states come from? Both physical illness and illness ascribed to evil influence, according to the Buddhist tradition, are caused fundamentally by the emotions that we call attachment, aversion, and indifference, which we referred to earlier as the three poisons. These emotions may eventually result in imbalances, and these imbalances in turn make us ill, both physically and mentally. This may be easier to accept if you carefully explore the different relationships among the elements of our minds and bodies based on cause and effect. Centuries of investigation by Tibetan physicians has located the source of different types of disease and evil influence within those basic negative emotions in different combinations,

---

* The Tibetan words for these three factors do not literally correlate with the English translations. Thus, the term "gall" should not be taken as meaning the fluid that is in the gallbladder, and "phlegm" does not literally mean the substance produced by diseased lungs.

and treatment of those diseases therefore takes place on both the mental and physical level. That is how Tibetan medicine explains disease.

To treat emotional disorders, a Tibetan doctor will give advice on how to alter the state of mind, or the attitude, of the sick person. The person could be feeling ill at ease due to intense anger or due to holding a strong grudge. There are certain psychological exercises that the sick person can do in order to diminish anger, and thereby alleviate the disorder. In such cases, the doctor will basically act as a therapist.

When a Tibetan doctor is faced with a patient, it's necessary to make a diagnosis. In Tibet there were no technological resources for making a diagnosis. The doctor relied on what was at hand. A Tibetan doctor utilizes two diagnostic approaches. One is checking subtle changes in the pulse at the wrist, and the other is examination of the urine. Through pulse diagnosis, a doctor can find out whether a patient has a normal illness, one due to evil influence, or a combination of the two, and which of the two is the most dominant. If a Tibetan doctor is very learned and experienced, he will not initially ask any questions of the patient. He'll first check the pulse, putting his three fingers over the pulse at the wrist, and spend some time checking the six subtle pulses that reflect conditions in different parts of the body. Then he will ask the patient, "Don't you suffer from such and such...?" If he's correct, he will be regarded as an experienced, valid doctor.

In urine diagnosis, the doctor observes the urine for different properties: its clarity, its color, how bubbles and foam are formed when stirring it, and the odor. From those observations, a variety of illnesses can be determined, based on the three factors I mentioned before—wind, gall, and phlegm—and their combinations.

In Tibetan medicine, the process of studying texts is not considered as important as the practical experience that comes after that. The best time for diagnosis is in the early morning, before the patient's body is agitated by activity. Then the diagnosis will be more precise. A truly expert Tibetan doctor can even detect how much of one's life-span is potentially remaining. That ability is very rare, however, even among Tibetan doctors.

The rest of the diagnostic process is probably similar to other coun-tries and other traditions. You check the face, the color of the face, the color of the eyes, how the eyes look, the nose, the tongue, skin tone, skin color, the posture, the breathing, the circulation, and so forth. The doctor takes advantage of all of these observable characteristics.

As mentioned, Tibetan medicine understands all disorders, physi-cal and mental, as ultimately manifestations of the three mind poisons: attachment, aversion, and indifference. The three mind poisons stem from ignorance, the lack of knowing of our true mind nature. From the Tibetan point of view, as long as ignorance has not been cleared up, there is no way to have perfect health. The main point is that if you want to be rid of disease, it is necessary to eliminate ignorance. If you want to remove the symptoms, you need to remove the causes. This is why they say that any ordinary sentient being by default cannot escape illness and evil influences: their minds are constantly under the influence of the three poisons.

So, we can understand that the root cause of illness is the three toxic emotions, and the root of these three is ignorance. Ignorance is a lack of knowing—not knowing the basic nature of things. Therefore, we need to come to know the basic nature—the unconditioned nature—of our minds, beyond clinging. We need more than a glimpse of this nature; we need to strengthen this experience to such an extent that it becomes stable. Once we are able to stabilize the experience of our own unconditioned nature, we become, by definition, free of illness and negative influences. An awakened being, a buddha, is sometimes described as having conquered the four demons. One of those demons is the disturbing emotions, which are the root cause of all illness.

When we become ill with a particular disease it is usually the result of some circumstance. From the point of view of Tibetan medicine, a group of circumstances converge to produce a state of illness. These circumstances include things such as place, time, temperature, attitude, and food. All these together can contribute to a certain kind of disorder. The external world we live in, the natural environment, consists of earth, water, fire, wind, and space. This physical body is correlated to those five elements—we have flesh, blood, temperature, breath, and air spaces within.

A certain balance is required in order to be at ease. In the past the weather and the environment were not so much on people's minds, but these days it seems to be an ever-present worry. Either there is too much water, or not enough. Too much heat, or not enough. When these factors become extreme, we begin to worry that we won't be able to live in a certain place. The whole world environment seems to be getting a little shaky. Why? Because of an imbalance of the external elements. In other words, the environment has gotten ill.

There is at least one good aspect, and that is that the environment is incapable of feeling and therefore doesn't suffer. The inhabitants of the environment, however, are alive and conscious and able to feel. When the environment is out of balance we feel uncomfortable. Among all the inhabitants of the environment, human beings are the most capable. We know how to shelter ourselves from too much heat, too much water, too much wind, and so forth. We know how to store nourishment for bad times. That's what human beings do, they think ahead and try to make themselves comfortable and safe. But there are other beings and animals who are not so capable of protecting themselves from environmental changes, and they suffer when there is a huge imbalance of heat, cold, or moisture. They don't have the ability to take care of themselves in changing situations. When it gets really difficult, animals suffer tremendously.

Like in the external world, imbalance in the body also causes suffering. In the internal environment, an imbalance of the three factors of wind, gall, and phlegm brings illness. Wind disorder can be provoked by a lot of different things, but mainly from mental worry or stress. Worrying and thinking too much can make a person sick. The other two disorders are mainly related to nutrition.

Wind disorders are often diagnosed as mental disorders, but they can be produced by external circumstances. A slight wind disorder is not such a big problem. One may have difficulty sleeping at night or feel nervous or unsettled for no apparent reason. That's not so difficult to deal with. It can be cured. If one has a stronger wind disorder, then one is described as mentally unstable, and if the imbalance is very strong, one is called insane. Drugs are prescribed in the Tibetan medical system, but drugs are not the primary factor in recovery. The environment the patient is put in has the biggest impact. It should be quiet and without anything that feels like a burden. There should be clean air, and the person should be able to see the sky. Removing sources of worry is the primary treatment. Wind disorder is something that any of us may have from time to time, not just some susceptible people.

The second type of disease is gall disorder. This does not refer to a specific disease of the gall bladder. It comes about by eating a diet that is too greasy, especially if the fat or the oil is old or rancid. Gall disorder makes the body feel heavy, and one feels depressed or irritable for no reason. Just as before, a doctor can prescribe certain behavior, environments, diet, and medicine. Most medicines for gall disorder are very bitter—they taste awful. Under this heading you also find descriptions of jaundice and other types of liver disorders, and in the Tibetan tradition these are not considered major problems. If they can be detected at the beginning, before the skin has turned yellow, there is medicine that can clear it up very fast. The Indian Ayurvedic tradition and the Tibetan tradition both have medicines to treat such symptoms. In the Tibetan medical tradition there is a very bitter drink that can clear up jaundice within five or six days. Another type of medicine for gall disorder consists of a drink made from sugar cane, not the sugar but the cane itself. It helps to remove more quickly the yellowness in the body after it has appeared.

The third type of disease is phlegm disorder. Once a phlegm disorder has grown chronic, it becomes very difficult to cure. There are many different variations of phlegm disorder, but they also require a particular diet, environment, behavior, and medicine. A cancerous disorder would be included under the phlegm type. Tibetan doctors have studied cancer over the last few decades, and they relate cancer to one of eighteen types of diseases called *nyen* in Tibetan. Of these eighteen diseases, some can be cured at the onset, but not after they start to spread through the body. Others of this category are incurable; it doesn't matter what you do. They attack and ruin specifically the vital organs, such as the spleen and the pancreas.

A skilled doctor will be able to detect the difference between a physical disorder and evil influence. If it's evil influence, medicine and drugs are not enough. Something else is necessary. In this situation certain rituals—ceremonies with mantras and chanting—are combined with a medical cure. For an emotional disorder, the doctor will give advice on how to change the state of mind, the attitude of the sick person. Intense anger or holding a strong grudge could be what is making the person ill at ease.

Among Tibetan healers there is the belief that a happy frame of mind is also a type of medicine for the sick person. How to put the patient at ease, how to make the person relax, is considered very important. To put the ill person at ease is a form of treatment. This relaxed frame of mind becomes the basis for subsequent treatment. Once the person is put at ease, then the medicine that is given in addition to that will not only work faster, but ultimately be more effective.

In the medical scriptures, some of which are more than one thousand years old and still in use today, there are clear descriptions of surgery, application of heat upon certain points of the body, and blood letting from different places. The instruments for these procedures still exist. However, the actual techniques for performing surgery, and therefore the ability to perform surgery, has died out. The texts describe abdominal surgery, the removal of cataracts, and other operations, but the tradition of performing this surgery no longer exists within Tibetan medicine. But they still use the application of heat to particular spots, and also of blood letting from particular points.

Blood letting is not a simple thing. One has to be very precise in determining the particular point of the body from which the diseased blood should be let out, how much blood, and which time of the day. The procedure needs to be done by an experienced doctor, otherwise it can be very dangerous. One needs to first distinguish between the diseased portion of the blood in the body, and the rest of the blood circulation, and make sure that only the diseased part comes out and the rest stays in.

There are certain disorders for which Tibetan medicine is particularly useful. One is the wind disorder, which manifests as feeling anxious, unsettled, or having difficulty sleeping. These are common complaints in Western patients as well, I believe. Bile disorder causes jaundice, but there are milder forms in which you just feel tired or sluggish for no reason. Tibetan medicines can help clear up both wind disorder and bile disorder.

Overall, there are three major ways of healing within the Tibetan medical tradition. The first method utilizes physical substances, medicines that can be taken internally. The second method uses mantra, certain phrases or sounds that are repeated many times. The third method relies on practice in achieving a state called *samadhi*, or relaxed contemplation accomplished through spiritual practice. The wisdom that the doctor achieves through spiritual practice can also help to heal the patient.

These last two methods may be a bit difficult for scientifically minded people to accept. However, I've heard that there is currently Western scientific research on the subject of whether prayer, performed on behalf of patients who don't even know they are being prayed for, can improve healing. The studies have so far shown a beneficial effect. There are also studies on Western people who were taught to meditate in which the function of their immune system showed measurable improvement. So it may be good to keep an open mind on this topic.

In Tibetan medicine there is the strong belief in the importance of the physician's noble intentions. This is in addition to the skill necessary to make a diagnosis and recommend treatment. If the doctor has a good heart, the medicine that is prescribed will be more effective. This is a very common belief in Tibet. In the Tibetan medical system, as in the Western medical system, the doctors have to be very smart, and learn a lot. The signs and symptoms of illness, and the appropriate treatments must all be memorized. In addition, Tibetan doctors often gather herbs and make their own medicines. A doctor may be very skillful and intelligent, doing everything properly, but if his or her attitude is too proud, then his or her loving-kindness and caring may be poor. As a result, the healing may be mediocre. In contrast, a doctor who is not particularly learned, but has an extremely good heart, may be able to to be more effective at healing people.

Ultimately, we judge a doctor, not just on their educational achievements, but also by how noble-minded the person is. It would be interesting to see from a Western scientific point of view whether you can measure a relationship between the doctor's good will and the effectiveness of that doctor's medical treatment—in other words, whether there is a detectable benefit from the good wishes and the energy of a compassionate doctor directed toward their patient. In Tibet, the benefit of this positive attitude is commonly accepted and is valued more than the medicine itself.

This is the key point of this whole book. Combining medicine and compassion means resolving to cultivate compassion—the will to ease suffering—in order to benefit your patients. Once that noble resolve is made, everything else will flow from that. Possessing a noble heart is very precious. It is the most important principle in healing.

Afterword

TRYING TO IMAGINE COMPASSION that can flow spontaneously from our basic nature, as Chokyi Nyima Rinpoche has described in this book, may seem impossible at first. Just remember, many Western scientific insights, such as the theory of relativity and quantum mechanics, are equally difficult to understand and accept when first described. Through reading and reflection, the ideas become more and more familiar and acceptable. However, at some point it may become necessary to find a teacher who can give advice on how you can train to recognize your own basic nature. In Buddhist philosophy, this type of training is always given in person. In this manner, a qualified teacher can steer the motivated student in just the right ways to make the jump from what at first seems conceptually impossible to something that has been personally experienced. At that point, further training reinforces the insight, making it more and more stable.

Many people have suggested to me that *Medicine and Compassion* should be directed to first- and second-year medical students. In fact, I think medical students would benefit greatly from this book (it would make a great present for anyone you know who is starting medical school). However, in order to allow students to truly grow in their compassion, the mentoring environment of the hospital also needs to gradually change to enable the students to gain confidence in their efforts. We need attending physicians who talk about compassion as easily as, say, cardiac failure. We need to shift the center of gravity in medical centers such that not being kind to patients is seen as a failing, whether one's diagnostic and treatment skills are exemplary or not.

For those of you who look at your already incredibly busy lives and wonder how you can find any additional time to read about and train in compassion, just remember Chokyi Nyima Rinpoche's advice: You always find time to do the things that you are truly interested in. As you become more and more interested in compassion and begin to feel the benefits of the efforts you have made, you will automatically find more time.

David R. Shlim, M.D.

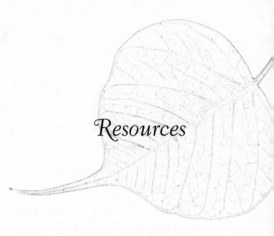

Resources

I F YOU HAVE BEEN INSPIRED by this book, but are wondering what to do next, here are some ideas. The ability to increase your capacity for compassion requires resources. Some of you may feel a connection with the words of Chokyi Nyima Rinpoche and want to experience more teachings from him. Chokyi Nyima Rinpoche resides in Kathmandu, Nepal, at the Ka-Nying Shedrup Ling Monastery. You can write to him at:

> Venerable Chokyi Nyima Rinpoche
> Ka-Nying Shedrup Ling Monastery
> PO Box 1200
> Boudhanath, Kathmandu
> Nepal
> E-mail: cn_rinpoche@yahoo.com

For those of you who would like to contact Dr. David Shlim, he resides in a small town outside of Jackson, Wyoming. His address is:

> David R. Shlim, M.D.
> P.O. Box 40
> Kelly, WY 83011
> E-mail: drshlim@wyom.net

Dr. Shlim would love to hear from readers of the book about how they responded to it. He would like to collect stories of compassion—and stories of overt lack of compassion—from the medical and caregiver world, and use these to encourage and promote the greater emphasis on compassion in medical care. Please e-mail or mail your stories to his address above.

Medicine and Compassion is part of a long-term project by Dr. Shlim and Chokyi Nyima Rinpoche to help establish the idea that compassion can be trained in and made more effortless, with great benefits to both patient and caregiver. To stay in touch with this project, and to find out about future seminars in Medicine and Compassion by Chokyi Nyima Rinpoche and others, you can visit our website:

www.medicineandcompassion.com

Chokyi Nyima Rinpoche plans to give a seminar on Medicine and Compassion in July 2005 in Boston, Massachusetts.

Chokyi Nyima Rinpoche is the spiritual head of the Chokling Tersar Foundation, whose aim is to preserve and promote authentic Tibetan Buddhist teachings in North America. Dr. Shlim is President of the Chokling Tersar Foundation. The foundation owns a sixty-acre retreat center in northern California where Chokyi Nyima Rinpoche gives seminars every summer. Each year the retreat center, called Gomde USA, also hosts a number of other qualified teachers within the Tibetan tradition. For more information on the activities of the Chokling Tersar Foundation, visit the website at: www.gomdeusa.org. The mailing address is:

Chokling Tersar Foundation
Rangjung Yeshe Gomde USA
66000 Drive Thru Tree Road
PO Box 162
Leggett, CA 95585-0162

Other Books by Chokyi Nyima Rinpoche

Chokyi Nyima Rinpoche is the author of several books in addition to *Medicine and Compassion,* including:

The Union of Mahamudra and Dzogchen (Rangjung Yeshe Publications) presents Chokyi Nyima Rinpoche's commentary on a classic Tibetan Buddhist text. The book walks the reader through a complete introduction to basic Tibetan Buddhist philosophy. It is an excellent follow-up to Medicine and Compassion for someone who would like to pursue the philosophic basis of Tibetan Buddhism in more detail.

The Bardo Guidebook (Rangjung Yeshe Publications) is Chokyi Nyima Rinpoche's commentary on a classic Tibetan Buddhist text called *The Mirror of Mindfulness. The Bardo Guidebook* gives clear and complete guidance on the four major stages in our lives and on how to maximize our potential at each stage. Particular attention is given to the stage between the time of dying and the time of taking rebirth.

Indisputable Truth (Rangjung Yeshe Publications). In this book, Rinpoche says: "All the 84,000 types of teachings given by our compassionate teacher Buddha Shakyamuni can be condensed into the Four Seals of the Dharma. In this book I will explain these four seals to the best of my ability."

Present Fresh Wakefulness (Rangjung Yeshe Publications). The subtitle of this book is *A Meditation Manual on Nonconceptual Wisdom.* The book explores ways to gain understanding of our basic nature, our "present fresh wakefulness."

Song of Karmapa (Rangjung Yeshe Publications). Chokyi Nyima Rinpoche writes in this book: "The message is simply that we should realize our basic wakefulness, our innate self-existing wisdom. We must receive instructions on how to remove the obscurations preventing realization of our own buddha nature. The essential substance expressed in Dharma teachings is really nothing more than this."

Chokyi Nyima Rinpoche also comments on the famous *Eight Verses of Mind Training* in his introduction to the recent book from Wisdom Publications, *Uniting Wisdom and Compassion: Illuminating the Thirty Seven Practices of Bodhisattvas.*

Suggested Further Reading

The Art of Happiness: A Handbook for Living by The Dalai Lama and Howard C. Cutler, M.D. A very user-friendly introduction to Tibetan Buddhist philosophy in the form of a dialogue between the author, who is a doctor, and the Dalai Lama.

A Beginner's Guide to Tibetan Buddhism by Bruce Newman (Snow Lion Publications, 2004). The book answers a lot of questions that arise as one begins to practice Tibetan Buddhism. The author's experience is based on his nearly thirty-year personal relationship with Chokyi Nyima Rinpoche.

Buddhist Himalayas by Olivier Follmi, Danielle Follmi, and Matthieu Ricard (Harry N. Abrams, 2002). A large format photographic portrait of Tibetan spiritual and everyday life, with an extraordinary collection of essays on Buddhist philosophy and life.

The Compassionate Life by The Dalai Lama (Wisdom Publications, 2003). Explores the connection between increasing your compassion and your sense of personal happiness.

The Tibetan Book of Living and Dying by Sogyal Rinpoche (Harper San Francisco 1992). An inspiring and accessible presentation of Tibetan Buddhist philosophy as it applies to the problems of everyday life.

Repeating the Words of the Buddha by Tulku Urgyen Rinpoche (Rangjung Yeshe Publications, 1991). Basic instruction from the father of Chokyi Nyima Rinpoche. Tulku Urgyen Rinpoche lived simply his whole life and spent over twelve years in solitary retreat. He was a renowned master of dzogchen meditation.

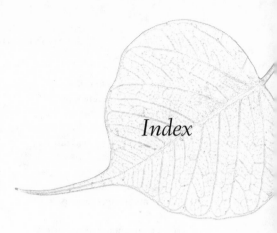

Index

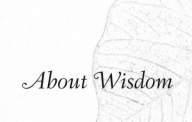

About Wisdom

WISDOM PUBLICATIONS, a nonprofit publisher, is dedicated to preserving and transmitting important works from all the major Buddhist traditions as well as related East-West themes.

To learn more about Wisdom, or browse our books on-line, visit our website at wisdompubs.org. You may request a copy of our mail-order catalog on-line or by writing to:

Wisdom Publications
199 Elm Street
Somerville, Massachusetts 02144 USA
Telephone: (617) 776-7416
Fax: (617) 776-7841
Email: info@wisdompubs.org
www.wisdompubs.org

The Wisdom Trust

As A NONPROFIT PUBLISHER, Wisdom is dedicated to the publication of fine books for the benefit of all sentient beings and dependent upon the kindness and generosity of sponsors in order to do so. If you would like to make a donation to Wisdom, please do so through our Somerville office. If you would like to sponsor the publication of a book, please write or email us at the address above.
Thank you.

Wisdom is a nonprofit 501(c)(3) organization affiliated with the Foundation for the Preservation of the Mahayana Tradition (FPMT).

41 one root of suffering is discontent = to know how to be content = happiness